CLINICAL COMPANION

D0557460

TENTH EDITION 10

FUNDAMENTALS of NURSING

Patricia A. Potter, RN, MSN, PhD, FAAN
Formerly, Director of Research
Patient Care Services
Barnes-Jewish Hospital
St. Louis, Missouri

Patricia A. Stockert, RN, BSN, MS, PhD
President, College of Nursing
Saint Francis Medical Center College of
  Nursing
Peoria, Illinois

Anne Griffin Perry, RN, EdD, FAAN
Professor Emerita
School of Nursing
Southern Illinois University-Edwardsville
Edwardsville, Illinois

Amy M. Hall, RN, BSN, MS, PhD, CNE
Dean, School of Nursing
Franciscan Missionaries of Our Lady
  University
Baton Rouge, Louisiana

ELSEVIER

Elsevier
3251 Riverport Lane
St. Louis, MO 63046

CLINICAL COMPANION FOR FUNDAMENTALS
OF NURSING, TENTH EDITION   ISBN: 978-0-323-71130-2

Notices

Practitioners and researchers must always rely on their own experience and
knowledge in evaluating and using any information, methods, compounds or
experiments described herein. Because of rapid advances in the medical sciences, in
particular, independent verification of diagnoses and drug dosages should be made.
To the fullest extent of the law, no responsibility is assumed by Elsevier, authors,
editors or contributors for any injury and/or damage to persons or property as a
matter of products liability, negligence or otherwise, or from any use or operation of
any methods, products, instructions, or ideas contained in the material herein.

Previous editions copyrighted 2017, 2013, 2009, 2005, 2001, 1997, 1993, 1989, and 1985.

Library of Congress Control Number: 2019949159

Director, Traditional Education: Tamara Myers
Senior Content Development Manager: Lisa Newton
Senior Content Development Specialist: Tina Kaemmerer
Publishing Services Manager: Deepthi Unni
Project Manager: Bharat Narang
Design Direction: Amy Buxton, Maggie Reid

Printed in the United States of America

Last digit is the print number: 9 8 7 6 5 4 3 2 1

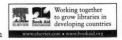

Preface

This *Clinical Companion* is a tool for quick reference of information critical to safe, patient-centered care. It provides resources for you to fulfill the Quality and Safety Education for Nurses (QSEN) and Institute of Medicine (IOM; now National Academy of Medicine [NAM]) competencies. It is a supplemental tool with condensed information from your *Fundamentals of Nursing* textbook.

This resource focuses on essential assessment and patient care information to guide your practice in nursing fundamentals, but you will also find it helpful for quick reference throughout your nursing program. It is a reference for use in class, lab, and clinical.

To pass your licensure exam and be prepared for nursing practice on graduation, you will need to have developed excellent clinical judgment skills while in your nursing program. Be sure to practice using the resources in this *Clinical Companion* to guide your development of those skills. Use the *Clinical Companion* as a reference while you work on case studies, practice communication and physical examination skills in the simulation lab or virtually, and care for patients in a variety of settings.

Contents

CHAPTER 1

Medical, Nursing, and Health Professions Terminology

ABBREVIATIONS

NOTE: Abbreviations in common use can vary widely. Each institution's list of acceptable abbreviations is the best authority for its records.

Abbreviation	Definition
ac	before meals
ACLS	advanced cardiac life support
ad lib	as desired
ADA	American Diabetes Association
ADD	attention deficit disorder
ADLs	activities of daily living
AIDS	acquired immunodeficiency syndrome
ALS	advanced life support; amyotrophic lateral sclerosis

Continued

Abbreviation	Definition
AM, am	morning
AMI	acute myocardial infarction
ASD	atrial septal defect
AST	aspartate aminotransferase (formerly SGOT)
A-V, AV, A/V	arteriovenous; atrioventricular
BCLS	basic cardiac life support
BE	barium enema
bid, b.i.d.	twice a day (bis in die)
BM	bowel movement
BMR	basal metabolic rate
BP	blood pressure
BPH	benign prostatic hypertrophy
bpm	beats per minute
BR	bed rest
BRP	bathroom privileges
BSA	body surface area
BSC	bedside commode
BSE	breast self-examination
BUN	blood urea nitrogen
Bx	biopsy
c̄	with
CABG	coronary artery bypass graft
CAD	coronary artery disease
CAT	computerized (axial) tomography scan
CBC, cbc	complete blood count
CCU	coronary care unit; critical care unit
CF	cystic fibrosis
CHD	congenital heart disease; coronary heart disease

Continued

Abbreviation	Definition
CHF	congestive heart failure
CK	creatinine kinase
CMV	cytomegalovirus
CNS	central nervous system
c/o	complaint of
CO	carbon monoxide; cardiac output
CO_2	carbon dioxide
COPD	chronic obstructive pulmonary disease
COX	cyclooxygenase
CP	cerebral palsy; cleft palate
CPAP	continuous positive airway pressure
CPK	creatine phosphokinase
CPR	cardiopulmonary resuscitation
CSF	cerebrospinal fluid
CT	computed tomography
CVA	cerebrovascular accident; costovertebral angle
CVP	central venous pressure
D&C	dilation (dilatation) and curettage
dc, DC, D/C	discontinue
DIC	disseminated intravascular coagulation
diff	differential blood count
DKA	diabetic ketoacidosis
DM	diabetes mellitus; diastolic murmur
DNA	deoxyribonucleic acid
DNR	do not resuscitate
DOA	dead on arrival
DOB	date of birth

Continued

Abbreviation	Definition
DOE	dyspnea on exertion
DPT	diphtheria-pertussis-tetanus
DRG	diagnosis-related group
DSM	*Diagnostic and Statistical Manual of Mental Disorders*
DT	delirium tremens
DVT	deep vein thrombosis
D_5W	dextrose 5% in water
Dx	diagnosis
EBV	Epstein-Barr virus
ECG, EKG	electrocardiogram; electrocardiograph
ECHO	echocardiography
ECT	electroconvulsive therapy
ED	emergency department
EDD	estimated date of delivery
EEG	electroencephalogram; electroencephalograph
EENT	eye, ear, nose, and throat
ELISA	enzyme-linked immunosorbent assay
EMG	electromyogram
EMS	emergency medical service
EMT	emergency medical technician
ENT	ear, nose, and throat
ER	emergency room (hospital)
ERV	expiratory reserve volume
ESR	erythrocyte sedimentation rate
ESRD	end-stage renal disease
ET	endotracheal tube
ETOH	ethyl alcohol
FBS	fasting blood sugar

Continued

Abbreviation	Definition
FEV	forced expiratory volume
FH, Fhx	family history
FHR	fetal heart rate
FOB	foot of bed
FTT	failure to thrive
fx	fracture
GB	gallbladder
GC	gonococcus; gonorrheal
GI	gastrointestinal
Grav I, II, etc.	pregnancy one, two, etc. (gravida)
GSW	gunshot wound
gtt	drops (guttae)
GU	genitourinary
Gyn	gynecology
H&P	history and physical
HA	headache
HAV	hepatitis A virus
Hb, HGB	hemoglobin
HBV	hepatitis B virus
HCG	human chorionic gonadotropin
HCT	hematocrit
HDL	high-density lipoprotein
HEENT	head, eye, ear, nose, and throat
HIV	human immunodeficiency virus
HOB, hob	head of bed
h/o	history of
HOH	hard of hearing
H_2O_2	hydrogen peroxide
HR, hr	heart rate; hour

Continued

Abbreviation	Definition
hs	bedtime
HSV	herpes simplex virus
HT, HTN, ht	hypertension; height
hx, Hx	history
I&O	intake and output
IBW	ideal body weight
ICP	intracranial pressure
ICU	intensive care unit
Ig	immunoglobulin
IM	intramuscular
INR	international normalized ratio
IUD	intrauterine device
IV	intravenous
IVP	intravenous pyelogram; intravenous push
IVPB	intravenous piggyback
KCl	potassium chloride
KUB	kidney, ureter, and bladder
KVO	keep vein open
L	liter
lab	laboratory
lb	pound
L&D	labor and delivery
LDL	low-density lipoprotein
LE	lower extremity; lupus erythematosus
LMP	last menstrual period
LOC	level of consciousness
LP	lumbar puncture
LR	lactated Ringer's
LVH	left ventricular hypertrophy

Continued

Abbreviation	Definition
MAP	mean arterial pressure
mcg	microgram
MD	muscular dystrophy
MDI	medium dose inhalant; metered dose inhaler
mEq	milliequivalent
mg	milligram
MI	myocardial infarction
mL, ml	milliliter
mm Hg	millimeters of mercury
MMR	maternal mortality rate; measles-mumps-rubella
MRI	magnetic resonance imaging
MVA	motor vehicle accident
N/A	not applicable
NaCl	sodium chloride
NANDA-I	North American Nursing Diagnosis Association–International
NAS	no added salt
N&V, N/V	nausea and vomiting
NG, ng	nasogastric
NICU	neonatal intensive care unit
NKA	no known allergies
NKDA	no known drug allergies
NPO, n.p.o.	nothing by mouth (non per os)
NSAID	nonsteroidal antiinflammatory drug
NSR	normal sinus rhythm
O_2	oxygen
OB	obstetrics
OBS	organic brain syndrome

Continued

Abbreviation	Definition
OOB	out of bed
OR	operating room
OTC	over-the-counter
oz	ounce
$\overline{p}$	after
PACU	postanesthesia care unit
PALS	pediatric advanced life support
pc	after meals
PCA	patient-controlled analgesia
PE	physical examination
PEEP	positive end-expiratory pressure
PERRLA	pupils equal, regular, react to light and accommodation
PET	positron emission tomography
PICC	percutaneously inserted central catheter
PID	pelvic inflammatory disease
PKU	phenylketonuria
PM, pm	evening
PMH	past medical history
PMI	point of maximal impulse
PMN	polymorphonuclear neutrophil leukocytes (polys)
PMS	premenstrual syndrome
PO, p.o.	orally (per os); by mouth
POD	postoperative day
PRN, p.r.n.	as required (pro re nata); as needed
pro time	prothrombin time
pt	pint
PT	prothrombin time; physical therapy

Continued

Abbreviation	Definition
PTT	partial thromboplastin time
PVC	premature ventricular contraction
q	every
qh	every hour
qid	four times a day
qt	quart
R	respiration; right; Rickettsia; roentgen
RBC, rbc	red blood cell; red blood count
RDA	recommended daily/dietary allowance
RDS	respiratory distress syndrome
Rh	rhesus factor in blood
RNA	ribonucleic acid
R/O	rule out
ROM	range of motion
ROS	review of systems
RR	recovery room; respiratory rate
R/T	related to
RX, Rx	prescription
s̄	without
SCD	sequential compression device
SGOT	serum glutamic oxaloacetic transaminase
SGPT	serum glutamic pyruvic transaminase
SIDS	sudden infant death syndrome
SLE	systemic lupus erythematosus
SOB	shortness of breath
S/P, s/p	status post
s/s	signs and symptoms
Staph	staphylococcus
stat	immediately (statim)

Continued

Abbreviation	Definition
STD	sexually transmitted disease
STI	sexually transmitted infection
Strep	streptococcus
Sx	symptoms
T	temperature; thoracic
T&A	tonsillectomy and adenoidectomy
TB	tuberculosis
TBL, tbsp, T	tablespoon
TENS	transcutaneous electrical nerve stimulation
TIA	transient ischemic attack
tid	three times a day
TMJ	temporomandibular joint
TPN	total parenteral nutrition
TPR	temperature, pulse, and respiration
TSE	testicular self-examination
TSH	thyroid-stimulating hormone
TSP, tsp, t	teaspoon
Tx	treatment
UA	urinalysis
URI	upper respiratory infection
UTI	urinary tract infection
VC	vital capacity
vol	volume
VS, v.s.	vital signs
VSD	ventricular septal defect
WBC, wbc	white blood cell; white blood count
WNL	within normal limits
WT, wt, wgt	weight

From *Mosby's dictionary of medicine, nursing, and health professions,* ed 10, St. Louis, 2017, Elsevier.

THE JOINT COMMISSION "DO NOT USE" LIST[1]

Do Not Use	Potential Problem	Use Instead
U, u (unit)	Mistaken for "0" (zero), the number "4" (four) or "cc"	Write "unit"
IU (International unit)	Mistaken for IV (intravenous) or the number 10 (ten)	Write "International unit"
Q.D., QD, q.d., qd (daily) Q.O.D., QOD, q.o.d, qod (every other day)	Mistaken for each other Period after the Q mistaken for "I" and the "O" mistaken for "I"	Write "daily" Write "every other day"
Trailing zero (X.0 mg)* Lack of leading zero (.X mg)	Decimal point is missed	Write X mg Write 0.X mg
MS MSO$_4$ and MgSO$_4$	Can mean morphine sulfate or magnesium sulfate Confused for one another	Write "morphine sulfate" Write "magnesium sulfate"

[1]Applies to all orders and all medication-related documentation that is handwritten (including free-text computer entry) or on preprinted forms.

*Exception: A "trailing zero" may be used only where required to demonstrate the level of precision of the value being reported, such as for laboratory results, imaging studies that report size of lesions, or catheter/tube sizes. It may not be used in medication orders or other medication-related documentation.

From The Joint Commission: *Facts about the official "Do Not Use" list of abbreviations,* 2018. https://www.jointcommission.org/facts_about_do_not_use_list/

INSTITUTE FOR SAFE MEDICATION PRACTICES (ISMP) LIST OF ERROR-PRONE ABBREVIATIONS AND SYMBOLS

The abbreviations, symbols, and dose designations found in this table have been reported to ISMP through the ISMP National Medication Errors Reporting Program (ISMP MERP) as being frequently misinterpreted and involved in harmful medication errors. They should **NEVER** be used when commu-

nicating medical information. This includes internal communications, telephone/verbal prescriptions, computer-generated labels, labels for drug storage bins, medication administration records, as well as pharmacy and prescriber computer order entry screens.

Abbreviations	Intended Meaning	Misinterpretation	Correction
μg	Microgram	Mistaken as "mg"	Use "mcg"
AD, AS, AU	Right ear, left ear, each ear	Mistaken as OD, OS, OU (right eye, left eye, each eye)	Use "right ear," "left ear," or "each ear"
OD, OS, OU	Right eye, left eye, each eye	Mistaken as AD, AS, AU (right ear, left ear, each ear)	Use "right eye," "left eye," or "each eye"
BT	Bedtime	Mistaken as "BID" (twice daily)	Use "bedtime"
cc	Cubic centimeters	Mistaken as "u" (units)	Use "mL"
D/C	Discharge or discontinue	Premature discontinuation of medications if D/C (intended to mean "discharge") has been misinterpreted as "discontinued" when followed by a list of discharge medications	Use "discharge" and "discontinue"
IJ	Injection	Mistaken as "IV" or "intrajugular"	Use "injection"
IN	Intranasal	Mistaken as "IM" or "IV"	Use "intranasal" or "NAS"
HS	Half-strength	Mistaken as bedtime	Use "half-strength" or "bedtime"
hs	At bedtime, hours of sleep	Mistaken as half-strength	
IU**	International unit	Mistaken as IV (intravenous) or 10 (ten)	Use "units"
o.d. or OD	Once daily	Mistaken as "right eye" (OD-oculus dexter), leading to oral liquid medications administered in the eye	Use "daily"
OJ	Orange juice	Mistaken as OD or OS (right or left eye); drugs meant to be diluted in orange juice may be given in the eye	Use "orange juice"
Per os	By mouth, orally	The "os" can be mistaken as "left eye" (OS-oculus sinister)	Use "PO," "by mouth," or "orally"
q.d. or QD**	Every day	Mistaken as q.i.d., especially if the period after the "q" or the tail of the "q" is misunderstood as an "i"	Use "daily"
qhs	Nightly at bedtime	Mistaken as "qhr" or every hour	Use "nightly"
qn	Nightly or at bedtime	Mistaken as "qh" (every hour)	Use "nightly" or "at bedtime"
q.o.d. or QOD**	Every other day	Mistaken as "q.d." (daily) or "q.i.d. (four times daily) if the "o" is poorly written	Use "every other day"
q1d	Daily	Mistaken as q.i.d. (four times daily)	Use "daily"
q6PM, etc.	Every evening at 6 PM	Mistaken as every 6 hours	Use "daily at 6 PM" or "6 PM daily"
SC, SQ, sub q	Subcutaneous	SC mistaken as SL (sublingual); SQ mistaken as "5 every;" the "q" in "sub q" has been mistaken as "every" (e.g., a heparin dose ordered "sub q 2 hours before surgery" misunderstood as every 2 hours before surgery)	Use "subcut" or "subcutaneously"
ss	Sliding scale (insulin) or ½ (apothecary)	Mistaken as "55"	Spell out "sliding scale;" use "one-half" or "½"
SSRI	Sliding scale regular insulin	Mistaken as selective-serotonin reuptake inhibitor	Spell out "sliding scale (insulin)"
SSI	Sliding scale insulin	Mistaken as Strong Solution of Iodine (Lugol's)	
i/d	One daily	Mistaken as "tid"	Use "1 daily"
TIW or tiw	3 times a week	Mistaken as "3 times a day" or "twice in a week"	Use "3 times weekly"
U or u**	Unit	Mistaken as the number 0 or 4, causing a 10-fold overdose or greater (e.g., 4U seen as "40" or 4u seen as "44"); mistaken as "cc" so dose given in volume instead of units (e.g., 4u seen as 4cc)	Use "unit"
UD	As directed ("ut dictum")	Mistaken as unit dose (e.g., diltiazem 125 mg IV infusion "UD" misinterpreted as meaning to give the entire infusion as a unit [bolus] dose)	Use "as directed"
Dose Designations and Other Information	**Intended Meaning**	**Misinterpretation**	**Correction**
Trailing zero after decimal point (e.g., 1.0 mg)**	1 mg	Mistaken as 10 mg if the decimal point is not seen	Do not use trailing zeros for doses expressed in whole numbers
"Naked" decimal point (e.g., .5 mg)**	0.5 mg	Mistaken as 5 mg if the decimal point is not seen	Use zero before a decimal point when the dose is less than a whole unit
Abbreviations such as mg. or mL. with a period following the abbreviation	mg mL	The period is unnecessary and could be mistaken as the number 1 if written poorly	Use mg, mL, etc. without a terminal period

Continued

Dose Designations and Other Information	Intended Meaning	Misinterpretation	Correction
Drug name and dose run together (especially problematic for drug names that end in "l" such as Inderal40 mg; Tegretol300 mg)	Inderal 40 mg Tegretol 300 mg	Mistaken as Inderal 140 mg Mistaken as Tegretol 1300 mg	Place adequate space between the drug name, dose, and unit of measure
Numerical dose and unit of measure run together (e.g., 10mg, 100mL)	10 mg 100 mL	The "m" is sometimes mistaken as a zero or two zeros, risking a 10- to 100-fold overdose	Place adequate space between the dose and unit of measure
Large doses without properly placed commas (e.g., 100000 units; 1000000 units)	100,000 units 1,000,000 units	100000 has been mistaken as 10,000 or 1,000,000; 1000000 has been mistaken as 100,000	Use commas for dosing units at or above 1,000, or use words such as 100 "thousand" or 1 "million" to improve readability

Drug Name Abbreviations	Intended Meaning	Misinterpretation	Correction
To avoid confusion, do not abbreviate drug names when communicating medical information. Examples of drug name abbreviations involved in medication errors include:			
APAP	acetaminophen	Not recognized as acetaminophen	Use complete drug name
ARA A	vidarabine	Mistaken as cytarabine (ARA C)	Use complete drug name
AZT	zidovudine (Retrovir)	Mistaken as azathioprine or aztreonam	Use complete drug name
CPZ	Compazine (prochlorperazine)	Mistaken as chlorpromazine	Use complete drug name
DPT	Demerol-Phenergan-Thorazine	Mistaken as diphtheria-pertussis-tetanus (vaccine)	Use complete drug name
DTO	Diluted tincture of opium, or deodorized tincture of opium (Paregoric)	Mistaken as tincture of opium	Use complete drug name
HCl	hydrochloric acid or hydrochloride	Mistaken as potassium chloride (The "H" is misinterpreted as "K")	Use complete drug name unless expressed as a salt of a drug
HCT	hydrocortisone	Mistaken as hydrochlorothiazide	Use complete drug name
HCTZ	hydrochlorothiazide	Mistaken as hydrocortisone (seen as HCT250 mg)	Use complete drug name
MgSO4**	magnesium sulfate	Mistaken as morphine sulfate	Use complete drug name
MS, MSO4**	morphine sulfate	Mistaken as magnesium sulfate	Use complete drug name
MTX	methotrexate	Mistaken as mitoxantrone	Use complete drug name
NoAC	novel/new oral anticoagulant	No anticoagulant	Use complete drug name
PCA	procainamide	Mistaken as patient controlled analgesia	Use complete drug name
PTU	propylthiouracil	Mistaken as mercaptopurine	Use complete drug name
T3	Tylenol with codeine No. 3	Mistaken as liothyronine	Use complete drug name
TAC	triamcinolone	Mistaken as tetracaine, Adrenalin, cocaine	Use complete drug name
TNK	TNKase	Mistaken as "TPA"	Use complete drug name
TPA or tPA	tissue plasminogen activator, Activase (alteplase)	Mistaken as TNKase (tenecteplase), or less often as another tissue plasminogen activator, Retavase (reteplase)	Use complete drug names
ZnSO4	zinc sulfate	Mistaken as morphine sulfate	Use complete drug name

Stemmed Drug Names	Intended Meaning	Misinterpretation	Correction
"Nitro" drip	nitroglycerin infusion	Mistaken as sodium nitroprusside infusion	Use complete drug name
"Norflox"	norfloxacin	Mistaken as Norflex	Use complete drug name
"IV Vanc"	intravenous vancomycin	Mistaken as Invanz	Use complete drug name

Symbols	Intended Meaning	Misinterpretation	Correction
ʒ	Dram	Symbol for dram mistaken as "3"	Use the metric system
ℳ	Minim	Symbol for minim mistaken as "mL"	
x3d	For three days	Mistaken as "3 doses"	Use "for three days"
> and <	More than and less than	Mistaken as opposite of intended; mistakenly use incorrect symbol; "< 10" mistaken as "40"	Use "more than" or "less than"
/ (slash mark)	Separates two doses or indicates "per"	Mistaken as the number 1 (e.g., "25 units/10 units" misread as "25 units and 110" units)	Use "per" rather than a slash mark to separate doses
@	At	Mistaken as "2"	Use "at"
&	And	Mistaken as "2"	Use "and"
+	Plus or and	Mistaken as "4"	Use "and"
°	Hour	Mistaken as a zero (e.g., q2° seen as q 20)	Use "hr," "h," or "hour"
Φ or ⌀	zero, null sign	Mistaken as numerals 4, 6, 8, and 9	Use 0 or zero, or describe intent using whole words

**These abbreviations are included on The Joint Commission's "minimum list" of dangerous abbreviations, acronyms, and symbols that must be included on an organization's "Do Not Use" list, effective January 1, 2004. Visit www.jointcommission.org for more information about this Joint Commission requirement.

© ISMP 2015. Permission is granted to reproduce material with proper attribution for internal use within healthcare organizations. Other reproduction is prohibited without written permission from ISMP. Report actual and potential medication errors to the ISMP National Medication Errors Reporting Program (ISMP MERP) via the Web at www.ismp.org or by calling 1-800-FAIL-SAF(E).

ISMP
INSTITUTE FOR SAFE MEDICATION PRACTICES
www.ismp.org

From Institute for Safe Medication Practices (ISMP): *List of error-prone abbreviations and symbols,* 2015. https://www.ismp.org/tools/errorproneabbreviations.pdf.

ROOTS

Root	Definition
aden/o	gland
adip/o, lip/o, steat/o	fat
albin/o, leuk/o, leuc/o	white
angi/o, vas/o	vessel
anter/o	front, before
arteri/o	artery
arthr/o	joint
audi/o	hearing
blast/o	embryonic
brachi/o	arm
bronch/o	airway
carcin/o	cancer
cardi/o	heart
cephal/o	head
cerebr/o, encephal/o	brain
cervic/o	neck
chol/e	bile, gall
cholecyct/o	gallbladder
chondr/o	cartilage
cirrh/o, jaund/o, xanth/o	yellow
cleid/o	clavicle
col/o	colon
colp/o	vagina
cost/o	rib
crani/o	skull
crypt/o	hidden

ROOTS—Cont'd

Root	Definition
cutane/o, dermat/o, derm/o	skin
cyan/o	blue
cyst/o	urinary bladder, cyst
cyt/o	cell
dactyl/o	finger or toe
elast/o	elastic
enter/o	intestines
erythem/o, erythr/o, rube/o	red
gastr/o	stomach or ventral
glomerul/o	glomerulus
gloss/o	tongue
gon/o	genitals
gynec/o, gyn/o	female
hem/o, hemat/o	blood
hepat/o	liver
hist/o	tissue
hol/o	entire, complete
home/o	like, similar
hydr/o	water, liquid, hydrogen
hypn/o	sleep
hyster/o, metr/o	uterus
idi/o	distinct, unknown
ile/o	ileum
ili/o	ilium, flank
irid/o	iris of the eye
kerat/o	horny substance, cornea
labi/o	lip, labial

Continued

ROOTS—Cont'd

Root	Definition
lact/o	milk, lactic acid
laryng/o	larynx
later/o	side or lateral
lith/o	stone
lymph/o	lymph
mamm/o, mast/o	breast
medi/o	middle
medull/o	medulla
melan/o	black, darkness
men/o	menses
menig/o	meninges
my/o	muscle
myel/o	spinal cord, marrow
myring/o	eardrum
nas/o, rhin/o	nose
necr/o	death
nephr/o	kidney
neur/o	nerve, nervous tissue
nucle/o	nucleus
ocul/o, ophthalm/o	eye
odont/o	teeth
onc/o	tumor, mass
onych/o	nail
oophor/o, ovari/o	ovary
orchid/o	testicle
oste/o	bone
ot/o	ear
path/o	disease
ped/o	foot, children

ROOTS—Cont'd

Root	Definition
phag/o	ingestion, eating
phleb/o	vein
pneum/o	air, breath
poster/o	behind, posterior
proct/o	anus, rectum
proxim/o	near
psych/o	mind, mental
py/o	pus
pyel/o	pelvis
pylor/o	pylorus
rachi/o	spine
radi/o	radioactive
ren/o	kidney
salping/o	tube
scler/o	hard
splen/o	spleen
squam/o	scale
thorac/o	chest, chest wall
thromb/o	blood clot
tox/o	poison
trache/o	trachea, windpipe
trich/o	hair
ur/o	urine
ureter/o	ureter
urethr/o	urethra
ventr/o	abdomen, ventral
vesic/o	bladder, vesicle
viscer/o	body organs

From Yoost BL, Crawford LR: *Fundamentals of nursing: active learning for collaborative practice*, ed 2, St. Louis, 2020, Elsevier.

PREFIXES

Prefix	Definition
a-	before, without
ab-	away from
acu-	clarity, sharpness
ad-	toward
all-, allo-	divergence
ambi-	both
an-	not, without
ante-	before
anti-	against
arch-, arche-, archi-	first, beginning
aur-, auro-	ear
auto-	self
bar-, baro-	weight, pressure
bi-, di-, diplo-	two, double
bili-	bile
bio-	life
brady-	slow
bucco-	cheek
caud-	tail
chemo-	chemical
circum-	around
co-	together
contra-, counter-	against
cryo-	cold
de-	from, removal
demi- hemi-, semi-	half

PREFIXES—Cont'd

Prefix	Definition
dia-	through
dis-	removal, separation
duct-	carry
dys-	abnormal, difficult, painful
ecto-	outside
endo-, ento-, im-, in-, intra-	within
epi-	upon, over
episio-	perineum
esthesi-	sensation, feeling
etio-	causation
eu-	normal, good, true
ex-	out
exo-	outside of
extra-	outside, in addition to
fasci-, fascio	fibrous membrane, band
fibro-	fibrous tissue
hetero-	other, different
homo-, homeo-	same
hyper-	high, increased, above
hypo-, sub-	under, decreased
iatro-	medicine, healing
immuno-	free from, immune
in-, im-	not
infra-, sub-	below, under
inter-	between
intra-	within
intro-	on the inside

Continued

PREFIXES—Cont'd

Prefix	Definition
iso-	equal, same
juxta-	near
macro-	large
mal-	bad, poor
megalo-	abnormally large
meso-	middle
meta-	beyond, over
micro-	abnormally small
mono-, uni-	one
multi-	many
neo-	new
nocto-	night
non-	not
oligo-	little
oo-	egg
ortho-	straight, correct
pan-	all
para-	beside, near
per-	by, through
peri-	around
poly	many
post-	after, behind
pre-, pro-	before, in front of
prim-	first
pseudo-	false
quad-	four
re-	back, again
retro-	backward, behind

PREFIXES—Cont'd

Prefix	Definition
super-	above, excessive
supra-	above
syn-, sym-	together
tachy-	fast
trans-	through, across
tri-	three
ultra-	beyond
un-	not

From Yoost BL, Crawford LR: *Fundamentals of nursing: active learning for collaborative practice,* ed 2, St. Louis, 2020, Elsevier.

SUFFIXES

Suffix	Definition
-ac, -al, -ary, -eal, -ic, -ory, -ous	pertaining to
-acro	extremity, extreme point
-agogue	producer, secretor
-agra	sudden, severe pain
-algia, dynia	pain
-ase	enzyme
-asis, -ia, -ism, -osis	condition
-asthenia	weakness
-ather, -athero	fatty plaque
-cardia	action of the heart
-cardio	heart
-cele	swelling, hernia
-centesis	puncture of a cavity

Continued

SUFFIXES—Cont'd

Suffix	Definition
-cide	destroying, killing
-clysis	washing, flushing
-crine	secrete
-crit	separate
-cyte	cell
-desis	binding, fixation
-ectasis	expansion, dilation
-ectomy	cutting out
-emia	blood condition
-form	in the shape of
-gen, -genic	produce, production
-gram	writing, record
-graph	instrument used to write or record
-graphy	process of writing or recording
-iatric	medicine
-ics	body of knowledge
-itis	inflammation
-lith	stone
-logy	study of
-lysis	dissolving, separating
-malacia	softening
-megaly	abnormal enlargement
-meter	measuring instrument
-metry	to measure
-odynia	pain
-oid	resembling
-ole, -ule	small
-oma	tumor

SUFFIXES—Cont'd

Suffix	Definition
-para	to bear, give birth
-pathy	disease, feeling
-penia	deficiency
-pexy	surgical fixation
-phagia	eating, ingestion
-phasia	speech
-philia, -phile, -philic	affinity for
-plasia	formation, molding
-plasty	plastic repair
-plegia	paralysis
-pnea	breathing
-poiesis	growth, formation
-rrhage, -rrhagia, -rrhagy	burst forth
-rrhaphy	surgical repair
-rrhea	flow, discharge
-rrhexis	rupture
-scope	instrument for viewing
-scopy	visual examination
-stasis	stoppage of flow
-stenosis	narrowing
-stomy	surgical opening
-tome, -tomy	cutting
-tripsy	crushing
-trophy	nutrition, growth
-tropia, -tropic	deviation from normal, have influence on
-uria	presence of a substance in urine

From Yoost BL, Crawford LR: *Fundamentals of nursing: active learning for collaborative practice*, ed 2, St. Louis, 2020, Elsevier.

For additional information on medical, nursing, and health professions terminology, consult the following:

Institute for Safe Medication Practices (ISMP) List of Error-Prone Abbreviations and Symbols, 2015. Retrieved from https://www.ismp.org/tools/errorproneabbreviations.pdf.

Leonard P: *Quick & Easy Medical Terminology,* ed 8, St. Louis, 2017, Elsevier

Mosby's dictionary of medicine, nursing & health professions, ed 10, St. Louis, 2017, Mosby.

Potter PA, Perry AG, Stockert PA, Hall AM: *Fundamentals of nursing*, ed 10, St. Louis, 2021, Elsevier.

The Joint Commission*: Facts about the Official "Do Not Use" List of Abbreviations*. Retrieved from https://www.jointcommission.org/facts_about_do_not_use_list/.

Yoost BL, Crawford LR: *Fundamentals of nursing: active learning for collaborative practice*, ed 2, St. Louis, 2020, Elsevier.

Yoost BL, Crawford LR: *Conceptual Care Mapping: case studies for improving communication, collaboration, and care,* St. Louis, 2018, Elsevier.

CHAPTER 2

Communication

VERBAL THERAPEUTIC COMMUNICATION TECHNIQUES

Technique	Examples	Rationale
Offering self	"I'll sit with you for a while." "I'll stay with you until your family member arrives."	• Demonstrates compassion and concern for the patient • Establishes a caring relationship
Calling the patient by name	"Good morning, Mr. Trimble." "Hi, Ms. Martin. How are you feeling this evening?"	• Conveys that the nurse sees the patient as an individual • Shows respect and helps to establish a caring relationship

Continued

VERBAL THERAPEUTIC COMMUNICATION TECHNIQUES— Cont'd

Technique	Examples	Rationale
Sharing observations	"You look tense." "You seem frustrated." "You are smiling."	• Raises the patient's awareness of his or her nonverbal behavior • Allows the patient to validate the nurse's perceptions • Provides an opening for the patient to share possible joys or concerns
Giving information	"It is time for your bath." "My name is Pam, and I will be the RN taking care of you until 7 p.m." "Your surgery is scheduled for 10:30 a.m. tomorrow."	• Informs the patient of facts needed in a specific situation • Provides a means to build trust and develop a knowledge base on which patients can make decisions

Continued

VERBAL THERAPEUTIC COMMUNICATION TECHNIQUES— Cont'd

Technique	Examples	Rationale
Using open-ended questions or comments	"What are some of your biggest concerns?" "Tell me more about your general health status." "Share some of the feelings you experienced after your heart attack."	• Gives the patient the opportunity to share freely on a subject • Avoids interjection of feelings or assumptions by the nurse • Provides for patient elaboration on important topics when the nurse wants to collect a breadth of information
Using focused questions or comments	"Point to exactly where your pain is radiating." "When did you start experiencing shortness of breath?" "How has your	• Encourages the patient to share specific data necessary for completing a thorough assessment • Asks the patient to provide details

Continued

VERBAL THERAPEUTIC COMMUNICATION TECHNIQUES— Cont'd

Technique	Examples	Rationale
	family responded to your being hospitalized?" "What is your greatest fear?" "Where were you when the symptoms started?" "Tell me where you live."	regarding various concerns • Focuses on the immediate needs of the patient
Providing general leads	"And then?" "Go on." "Tell me more."	• Encourages the patient to keep talking • Demonstrates the nurse's interest in the patient's concerns
Conveying acceptance	"Yes." Nodding. "I follow what you are saying." "Uh huh."	• Acknowledges the importance of the patient's thoughts, feelings, and concerns
Using humor	"You are really walking well this morning."	• Provides encouragement

Continued

VERBAL THERAPEUTIC COMMUNICATION TECHNIQUES— Cont'd

Technique	Examples	Rationale
	I'm going to have to run to catch up!"	• May lighten heavy moments of discussion • Used properly, allows a patient to focus on positive progress or better times and does not change the subject of a conversation
Verbalizing the implied	*Patient:* "I can't talk to anyone about this." *Nurse:* "Do you feel that others won't understand?"	• Encourages a patient to elaborate on a topic of concern • Provides an opportunity for the patient to articulate more clearly a complicated topic or feeling that could be easily misunderstood

Continued

VERBAL THERAPEUTIC COMMUNICATION TECHNIQUES—Cont'd

Technique	Examples	Rationale
Paraphrasing or restating communication content	*Patient:* "I couldn't sleep last night." *Nurse:* "You had trouble sleeping last night?"	• Encourages patients to describe situations more fully • Demonstrates that the nurse is listening
Reflecting feelings or emotions	"You were angry when your surgery was delayed?" "You seem excited about going home today."	• Focuses on the patient's identified feelings based on verbal or nonverbal cues
Seeking clarification	"I don't quite follow what you are saying." "What do you mean by your last statement?"	• Encourages the patient to expand on a topic that may be confusing or that seems contradictory
Summarizing	"There are three things you are upset about: your family being too busy,	• Reduces the interaction to three or four points identified by

Continued

VERBAL THERAPEUTIC COMMUNICATION TECHNIQUES— Cont'd

Technique	Examples	Rationale
	your diet, and being in the hospital too long."	the nurse as being significant • Allows the patient to agree or add additional concerns
Validating	"Did I understand you correctly that...?"	• Allows clarification of ideas that the nurse may have interpreted differently than intended by the patient

NONVERBAL THERAPEUTIC COMMUNICATION TECHNIQUES

Technique	Examples	Rationale
Active listening	• Maintaining intermittent eye contact • Matching eye levels • Attentive posturing • Facing the patient • Leaning toward the person who is speaking • Avoiding distracting body movement	• Conveys interest in the patient's needs, concerns, or problems • Provides the patient with undivided attention • Sends a clear message of concern and interest
Silence	• Being present with a person without verbal communication	• Provides the patient time to think or reflect • Communicates concern when there is really nothing adequate to say in difficult or challenging situations
Therapeutic touch	• Holding the hand of a patient • Providing a back rub • Touching a patient's arm lightly • Shaking hands with a patient in isolation	• Conveys empathy • Provides emotional support, encouragement, and personal attention • Relaxes the patient

NONTHERAPEUTIC COMMUNICATION

Action	Examples	Rationale
Asking "why" questions	"Why did you do that?" "Why are you feeling that way?" "Why do you continue to smoke when you know it is unhealthy?"	• Implies criticism • May make the patient defensive • Tends to limit conversation • Requires justification of actions • Focuses on a problem rather than a possible solution
Using closed-ended questions or comments	"Do you feel better today?" "Did you sleep well last night?" "Have you made a decision about radiation yet?" "Are you ready to take your bath?" "Will you let me give you your medicine now?"	• Results in short, one-word, yes or no responses • Limits elaboration or discussion of a topic • Allows patient to refuse important care • Differs from focused questions that direct an interview

Changing the subject	Patient: "I'm having a difficult time talking with my daughter." Nurse: "Do you have grandchildren?" Patient: "I just want to die." Nurse: "Did you sleep well last night?"	• Avoids exploration of the topic raised by the patient • Demonstrates the nurse's discomfort with the topic introduced by the patient
Giving false reassurance	"Everything will be okay." "Surgery is nothing to be concerned about." "Don't worry; everything will be fine."	• Discounts the patient's feelings • Cuts off conversation about legitimate concerns of the patient • Demonstrates a need by the nurse to "fix" something that the patient just wants to discuss
Giving advice	"If it were me, I would…" "You should really exercise more." "You should absolutely have chemotherapy to treat your breast cancer if you expect to live."	• Discourages the patient from finding an appropriate solution to a personal problem

Continued

NONTHERAPEUTIC COMMUNICATION—Cont'd

Action	Examples	Rationale
	"Of course you should tell your coworkers that you've been diagnosed with cancer."	• Tends to limit the patient's ability to explore alternative solutions to issues that need to be faced • Implies a lack of confidence in the patient to make a healthy decision • Removes the decision-making authority from the patient
Giving stereotypical or generalized responses	"It's for your own good." "Keep your chin up." "Don't cry over spilt milk." "You will be home before long."	• Discounts patient feelings or opinions • Limits further conversation on a topic • May be perceived as judgmental
Showing approval or disapproval	"That's good." "You have no reason to be crying."	• Limits reflection by the patient • Stops further discussion on patient decisions or actions • Implies a need for patients to have the nurse's support and approval

Showing agreement or disagreement	"That's right." "I disagree with what you just said."	• Discontinues patient reflection on an introduced topic • Implies a lack of value for patient's thoughts, feelings, or concerns
Engaging in excessive self-disclosure or comparing the experiences of others	"I had the same type of cancer 2 years ago." "I have several family members who drink too much, too." "I go to that restaurant every Friday for fish."	• Implies that experiences related to a disease process are similar for all patients • Takes the focus away from the patient • Limits further reflection or problem solving by the patient
Comparing patient experiences	"The lady in room 250 just had this surgery last week and did just fine." "My uncle had this type of inflammatory bowel disease and ended up having to have a colostomy."	• Removes the focus of conversation from the patient • Invalidates each individual patient experience as being unique and important • Breaches confidentiality

Continued

NONTHERAPEUTIC COMMUNICATION—Cont'd

Action	Examples	Rationale
Using personal terms of endearment	"Honey." "Sweetie, it is time to take your medicine." "Sport, how about if you show me how well you can walk across the room?"	• Demonstrates disrespect for the individual • Diminishes the dignity of a unique patient • May indicate that the nurse did not take the time or care enough to learn or remember the patient's name
Being defensive	"The nurses here work very hard." "Your doctor is extremely busy." "This is the best hospital in the area." "You won't get any better care anywhere else."	• Moves the focus from the patient • Discounts the patient's feelings and thoughts on a subject • Limits further conversation on a topic of patient concern

From Yoost BL, Crawford LR: *Fundamentals of nursing: active learning for collaborative practice,* ed 2, St. Louis, 2020, Elsevier.

DEFENSE MECHANISMS

Defense Mechanism	Definition
Compensation	Using personal strengths or abilities to overcome feelings of inadequacy
Denial	Refusing to admit the reality of a situation or feeling
Displacement	Transferring emotional energy away from an actual source of stress to an unrelated person or object
Introjection	Taking on certain characteristics of another individual's personality
Projection	Attributing undesirable feelings to another person
Rationalization	Denying true motives for an action by identifying a more socially acceptable explanation
Regression	Reverting to behaviors consistent with earlier stages of development
Repression	Storing painful or hostile feelings in the unconscious, causing them to be temporarily forgotten
Sublimation	Rechanneling unacceptable impulses into socially acceptable activities
Suppression	Choosing not to think consciously about unpleasant feelings

From Yoost BL, Crawford LR: *Fundamentals of nursing: active learning for collaborative practice,* ed 2, St. Louis, 2020, Elsevier.

COMMUNICATION IN SPECIAL CIRCUMSTANCES

Hearing Impaired

- Encourage individuals who normally wear hearing aids to place them in their ears during morning care.
- Check or replace hearing aid batteries regularly to avoid most associated mechanical difficulties.
- Make sure areas for interaction are well lit with as little background noise as possible.
- Stay within 3 to 6 feet of hearing-impaired patients while conversing.
- Raise voice level slightly.
- Face the hearing-impaired person, and avoid turning away.
- Speak clearly.
- Contact a sign language interpreter to assist with communication of critical information.
- Use written communication on a whiteboard or tablet when providing or reinforcing detailed information.

Sign Language

Manual alphabet

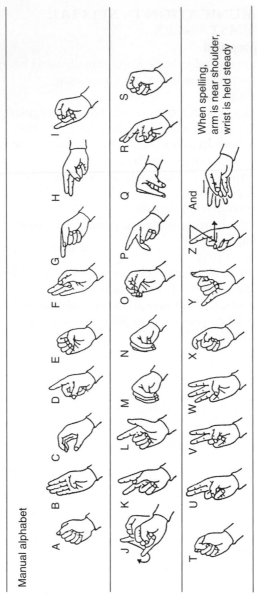

When spelling, arm is near shoulder, wrist is held steady

Numbers

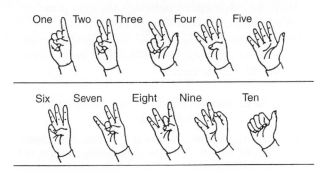

Visually Impaired
- Announce your arrival and/or tell the visually impaired person who you are when beginning interaction.
- Alert visually impaired patients of potential hazards or object locations.
- Use the analog clock position to describe the location of food on a plate or tray or the location of objects in a room.
- Access large-print, Braille, audio, or e-books as needed.
- Gently touch visually impaired patients on the arm if they are sleeping or if the environment is noisy before initiating interaction.

Physically or Cognitively Impaired
- Head nods, physical touch, or hand squeezes may be used to assist with communication.
- Whiteboards or tablets may facilitate communication based on individual needs.
- Utilize eye movement technology or electronic transducers when indicated.

- Observe nonverbal signs for indications of discomfort or needs.
- Adapt to a demented patient's thought process rather than confrontation or correction.

From Yoost BL, Crawford LR: *Fundamentals of nursing: active learning for collaborative practice,* ed 2, St. Louis, 2020, Elsevier.

For additional information on communication, consult the following:

Balzer Riley J: *Communication in Nursing,* ed 8, St. Louis, 2017, Elsevier.
Potter PA, Perry AG, Stockert PA, Hall AM: *Fundamentals of nursing,* ed 10, St. Louis, 2021, Elsevier.
Yoost BL, Crawford LR: *Conceptual Care Mapping: case studies for improving communication, collaboration, and care,* St. Louis, 2018, Elsevier.
Yoost BL, Crawford LR: *Fundamentals of nursing: active learning for collaborative practice,* ed 2, St. Louis, 2020, Elsevier.

CHAPTER 3

Interprofessional Collaboration and Delegation

INTERPROFESSIONAL COLLEAGUES

Health Care Team Members and Their Roles	Role of the Registered Nurse in Collaboration or Delegation
Primary care providers (PCPs): provide medical care, including diagnosing, treating, and preventing disease; may be a physician or nurse practitioner	Collaborates with PCPs to enhance patient well-being and care and promote positive patient outcomes
Medical specialist physicians: provide medical care for patients with diseases	Consults medical specialist physicians when providing specialized care for

Continued

INTERPROFESSIONAL COLLEAGUES—Cont'd

Health Care Team Members and Their Roles	Role of the Registered Nurse in Collaboration or Delegation
and disorders within their specialty	specific diseases and disorders
Surgical specialist physicians: perform diagnostic, ablative, constructive, reconstructive, transplantation, palliative, or cosmetic surgeries and procedures	Works together with surgical specialist physicians during the preoperative, intraoperative, and postoperative periods to provide patient care and monitor patient progress
Registered nurses (RNs): coordinate, direct, supervise, and provide patient care and patient education	Works cooperatively with other registered nurses to coordinate care for groups of patients and with specialized nurses, such as wound ostomy care nurses (WOCN), when necessary
Counselors: help patients cope with physical, emotional, psychological, or social issues	Works in partnership with counselors when patients need extra emotional or mental health support with issues surrounding their illness or situation
Dieticians: use knowledge of food	Refers patients to dieticians for nutritional

INTERPROFESSIONAL
COLLEAGUES—Cont'd

Health Care Team Members and Their Roles	Role of the Registered Nurse in Collaboration or Delegation
and nutrition to enhance patient wellness, healing, and recovery	support while addressing medical or surgical conditions, such as hypertension, dysphagia, or diabetes
Social workers: evaluate the patient's financial situation, support system, and home environment and determine availability of resources	Confers with social workers to determine hospitalization and home care coverage, as well as community referrals for home care needs
Unlicensed assistive personnel (UAP): perform direct patient care as delegated by the RN	Delegates to the UAP when patients require direct personal care and assistance with bathing, toileting, mobility, etc. UAPs are delegated to and supervised by the RN.
Laboratory technicians: collect and perform tests on samples of body fluids and tissues	Requests laboratory technicians to obtain and test samples for ordered laboratory tests
Pharmacists: prepare and dispense medications and IV fluids	Collaborates with pharmacists to obtain the correct ordered medications and IVs for each patient in the correct dosage

Continued

INTERPROFESSIONAL COLLEAGUES—Cont'd

Health Care Team Members and Their Roles	Role of the Registered Nurse in Collaboration or Delegation
Spiritual advisors (clergy, priests, ministers, rabbis, imams, etc.): counsel patients on spiritual matters and provide emotional support	Turns to spiritual advisors to provide spiritual support for ill and dying patients and their families
Licensed practical/ vocational nurses (LPNs/LVNs): provide direct patient care, including medication administration, wound care, and vital signs	Depends on LPNs/LVNs to provide patient care, perform treatments and administer oral medications and some IV medications depending on the training of the LPN/LVN
Speech pathologists and audiologists: evaluate and treat speech, language, hearing, swallowing, and communication disorders in patients	Consults speech pathologists and audiologists for assessment and interventions in patients with swallowing or speech deficits
Respiratory therapists: treat patients with diseases of the cardiopulmonary system and administer respiratory medications and treatments	Works in partnership with respiratory therapists to administer ordered respiratory medications to patients

INTERPROFESSIONAL COLLEAGUES—Cont'd

Health Care Team Members and Their Roles	Role of the Registered Nurse in Collaboration or Delegation
Physical therapists: evaluate and treat patients with mobility deficits	Joins forces with physical therapists to assess mobility, crutch walking, or walker stability or to provide rehabilitation for postsurgical or postinjury patients
Occupational therapists: evaluate activities of daily living (ADLs) and rehabilitate patients with deficits that affect ADLs and occupational tasks	Collaborates with occupational therapists to evaluate and care for patients with deficits in ADLs

PROFESSIONAL WEBSITES

For more information about the educational backgrounds and practice guidelines of health care team members with whom nurses collaborate, visit their professional organizations' websites.

Registered Dietitians
   www.nal.usda.gov/fnic/dietetic-associations
Physical therapists
   www.apta.org
Occupational therapists
   www.aota.org
Speech pathologists and audiologists
   www.asha.org
Social workers
   www.socialworkers.org/

Physicians
   www.ama-assn.org/ama
Pharmacists
   www.pharmacist.com
   Adapted from Yoost BL, Crawford LR: *Conceptual care mapping: case studies for improving communication, collaboration, and care*, St. Louis, 2018, Elsevier.

RIGHTS OF DELEGATION

1. *Right task:* one that is delegable for a specific patient
2. *Right circumstances:* appropriate patient setting, available resources, and other relevant factors considered
3. *Right person:* the right person delegating the right task to the right person to be performed on the right patient
4. *Right direction or communication:* clear, concise description of the task, including its objective, limits, and expectations
5. *Right supervision:* appropriate monitoring, evaluation, intervention, and feedback

TASKS THAT CAN AND CANNOT BE DELEGATED

Interventions That Can Be Delegated Following the Five Rights of Delegation	Interventions That Cannot Be Delegated
• Routine vital sign assessment of stable patients • Hygenic care such as bathing, shampooing, oral cleansing, and bed making • Back massage	• Assessment • Care planning • Development of a patient teaching plan • Changing dressings on acute wounds • Irrigating a wound

TASKS THAT CAN AND CANNOT BE DELEGATED—Cont'd

Interventions That Can Be Delegated Following the Five Rights of Delegation	Interventions That Cannot Be Delegated
• Toileting • Turning and positioning of patients • Range-of-motion exercises • Assistance with ambulation • Application of antiembolism hose or sequential compression devices • Changing a simple nonsterile dressing on an established wound in some facilities • Application of wraps, bandages, or binders • Collecting sputum, stool, and voided urine specimens • Blood glucose testing • Oral and oropharyngeal suctioning • Care of an established tracheostomy • Changing the pouch, or care of an ostomy without complications	• Collecting a wound culture or a urine specimen from a catheter • Tracheostomy, nasotracheal, or nasopharyngeal suctioning of a patient • Care of a new tracheostomy • Care of chest tubes • Changing the pouch of a new ostomy, or care of an ostomy with complications • Inserting a Foley catheter • Bladder irrigation • Medication administration • Starting and maintaining a peripheral IV • Patient education • Discharge instructions

From Yoost BL, Crawford LR: *Conceptual care mapping: case studies for improving communication, collaboration, and care,* St. Louis, 2018, Elsevier.

For additional information on interprofessional collaboration and delegation, consult the following:

Potter PA, Perry AG, Stockert PA, Hall AM: *Fundamentals of nursing*, ed 10, St. Louis, 2021, Elsevier.

Sullivan M, Kiovsky R, Mason D, et al: Interprofessional collaboration and education, *Am J Nurs* 115(3):47–54, 2015.

Yoost BL, Crawford LR: *Conceptual care mapping: case studies for improving communication, collaboration, and care,* St. Louis, 2018, Elsevier.

Yoost BL, Crawford LR: *Fundamentals of nursing: active learning for collaborative practice*, ed 2, St. Louis, 2020, Elsevier.

CHAPTER 4

Nursing Process and Care Planning

NURSING PROCESS
- The nursing process is similar to the scientific process.
- It is dynamic, organized, collaborative, and universally adaptable for use in all types of health care settings.
- Nurses use critical thinking and clinical decision-making skills to adapt patient plans of care using the nursing process as a patient's or group's conditions or concerns change.

ASSESSMENT
- Assessment data can be collected from a variety of sources including the following:
  - Patients
  - Family members
  - Friends
  - Communities
  - Health care professionals

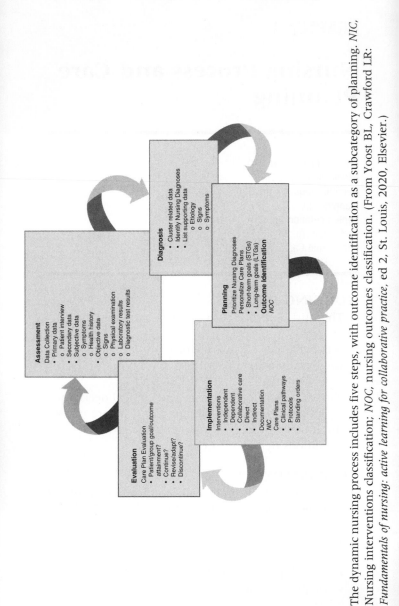

The dynamic nursing process includes five steps, with outcome identification as a subcategory of planning. *NIC,* Nursing interventions classification; *NOC,* nursing outcomes classification. (From Yoost BL, Crawford LR: *Fundamentals of nursing: active learning for collaborative practice,* ed 2, St. Louis, 2020, Elsevier.)

- Medical records
- Laboratory and diagnostic test results
- **S**ubjective data (symptoms) is **s**poken.
  - Stated feelings about a situation or condition
  - Difficult to validate
- **O**bjective data (signs) is **o**bservable information that the nurse gathers based on what can be seen, measured, or tested.
  - Medical record entries
  - Laboratory and diagnostic test results
  - Physical assessment findings

NURSING DIAGNOSIS

- Nursing diagnoses label patient or group.
  - Health problems
  - Potential concerns
  - Wellness initiative
- Nursing diagnostic labels are available from three primary taxonomies (unified language classification systems).
  - NANDA-I
  - International Classification for Nursing Practice (ICNP)
  - Clinical Care Classification (CCC) System

PLANNING

- Planning involves:
  - Prioritizing patient or group nursing diagnoses
  - Establishing short- and long-term goals
  - Choosing outcome indicators
  - Identification of interventions to address each specific goal

Maslow's Hierarchy of Needs

- Maslow's hierarchy of needs is helpful in prioritizing patient needs during the planning process.

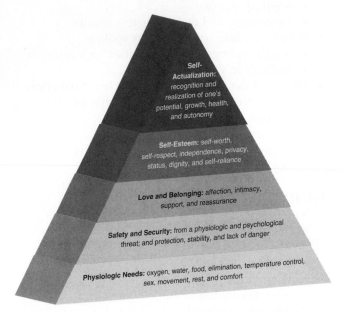

(From Yoost BL, Crawford LR: *Fundamentals of nursing: active learning for collaborative practice,* ed 2, St. Louis, 2020, Elsevier.)

Maslow's Hierarchy of Needs Applied to Patient Data

Level of Needs	Examples of Data
Physiologic: basic survival needs	Airway patency, breathing, circulation, oxygen level, nutrition, fluid intake, body temperature regulation, warmth, elimination, shelter, sexuality, infection, pain level

Maslow's Hierarchy of Needs Applied to Patient Data—Cont'd

Level of Needs	Examples of Data
Safety and security: need to be safe and comfortable	Physical safety (falls and drug side effects), psychological security (knowledge of routines and procedures, bedtime rituals, fear of isolation, and dependence needs)
Love and belonging: need for love and affection	Compassion of care provider, information from family and significant others, strength of support system
Self-esteem: need to feel good about oneself	Changes in body image (injury, surgery, puberty), changes in self-concept (ability to perform usual role functions), pride in abilities
Self-actualization: need to fulfill maximum potential; need for growth and change	Goal attainment, autonomy, motivation, problem-solving abilities, ability to provide and accept help, feeling of accomplishment, desired roles

From Yoost BL, Crawford LR: *Fundamentals of nursing: active learning for collaborative practice*, ed 2, St. Louis, 2020, Elsevier.

IMPLEMENTATION

- Implementation is the step during which nursing interventions or collaborative interventions are initiated or sustained.
- Evidence-based practice standards should be met to elicit the best possible patient or group outcomes.

- Evidence-based practice integrates:
  - Best research evidence
  - Clinical expertise of the nurse or primary care provider
  - Patient values and needs
  - Delivery of quality, cost-effective health care.

EVALUATION

- Evaluation focuses on the patient or group and the patient's or group's response to nursing interventions, and goal or outcome attainment.
- Evaluation identifies the effectiveness of implemented interventions.
- Evaluation must address:
  - Whether the goal/desired outcome (NOC) was met
  - Patient or group evidence of its achievement
  - If the plan of care should be continued, revised, or discontinued

CONCEPTUAL CARE MAPPING

- Conceptual care mapping is a contemporary method to develop dynamic plans of care.
- Conceptual care maps:
  - Mimic the thought process of the professional nurse while increasing his or her ability to accurately:
    - collect,
    - analyze, and
    - synthesize patient or group data
  - Guide patient care
  - Provide a tool for evaluation
- Conceptual care maps are a visual resource for developing and adapting plans of care online or in print.
- The CCM Creator is available as a resource with Yoost & Crawford's *Fundamentals of nursing: Active learning for collaborative practice,* ed 2, on the Evolve website.

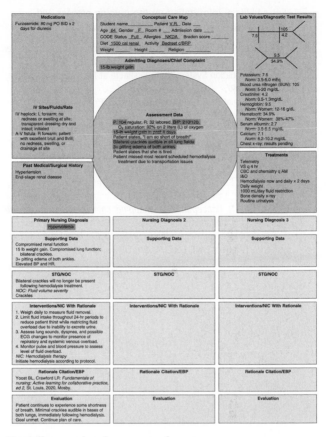

Partially completed conceptual care map.
EBP, Evidence-based practice; *ECG*, electrocardiogram; *IV*, intravenous; *NIC*, nursing interventions classification; *NOC*, nursing outcomes classification; *STG*, short-term goal.
(From Yoost B, Crawford, L: *Fundamentals of nursing: active learning for collaborative practice,* ed 2, St. Louis, 2020, Elsevier.)

For additional information on the nursing process and
care planning, consult the following:

Bulechek G, Butcher H, Dochterman J, Wagner C (eds): *Nursing interventions classifications (NIC)*, ed 7, St. Louis, 2018, Elsevier.

Clinical Care Classification System (CCC) available at https://www.sabacare. com/framework/.

International Classification for Nursing Practice (ICNP) available at https:// www.icn.ch/icnp-browser.

Moorhead S, Johnson M, Maas M, Swanson E: *Nursing outcomes classifi- cation (NOC)*, ed 6, St. Louis, 2018, Elsevier.

NANDA International, Inc.: *Nursing Diagnoses: Definitions and classification 2018-2020*, ed 11, New York, 2018, Thieme.

Potter PA, Perry AG, Stockert PA, Hall AM: *Fundamentals of nursing*, ed 10, St. Louis, 2021, Elsevier.

Yoost BL, Crawford LR: *Conceptual Care Mapping: case studies for improving communication, collaboration, and care*, St. Louis, 2018, Elsevier.

Yoost BL, Crawford LR: *Fundamentals of nursing: active learning for collab- orative practice*, ed 2, St. Louis, 2020, Elsevier.

CHAPTER 5

Documentation

DOCUMENTATION

Effective Documentation

- Is factual and accurate
- Is complete but concise
- Is completed in a timely manner
- Uses proper grammar and spelling
- Uses standard abbreviations and proper medical terminology
- Is organized according to facility policy

Documentation Formats

- Source-oriented format: gives each profession a separate section of the record in which to do narrative charting.
- Problem-oriented medical record (POMR) integrates charting from the entire care team in the same section of the record. Several problem-oriented medical record formats follow.

Format	Elements
PIE	Problem, intervention, evaluation
APIE	Assessment, problem, intervention, evaluation
SOAP	Subjective data, objective data, assessment, plan
SOAPIE	Subjective data, objective data, assessment, plan, intervention, evaluation
SOAPIER	Subjective data, objective data, assessment, plan, intervention, evaluation, revisions to plan
DAR	Data, action, response
CBE	Charting by exception

From Yoost BL, Crawford LR: *Fundamentals of nursing: active learning for collaborative practice,* ed 2, St. Louis, 2020, Elsevier.

ELECTRONIC HEALTH RECORD

- The electronic health record (EHR) includes documentation over time from inpatient and outpatient electronic medical records.
- The electronic medical record (EMR) records one episode of care (an office visit or a hospitalization).
- Major components of the EHR are health information, diagnostic test results, an order-entry system, and decision support.
- Physicians, nurse practitioners, nurses, medical assistants, physician assistants, unlicensed assistive personnel (UAP), social workers, and therapists may contribute to the EHR.
- Nursing documentation includes all steps of the nursing process.
- Standardized language is used when documenting.

- Laboratory data and other test results are available in multiple care settings to facilitate making decisions regarding patient care.
- In some circumstances, documentation of care, including obtaining vital signs on stable patients and assisting with activities of daily living, may be delegated to the UAP.
- Registered nurses are responsible for reviewing documentation by UAP for all patients under their care.
- The EMR is the legal documentation of care provided to a patient.
- In the event of litigation, the medical record is often the only available evidence of the event in question.
- Medical record documentation should be based on fact, not opinions, and should be clear, concise, and timely.
- Every entry in a medical record must include a date, time, and signature with credentials.
- Ethical practice dictates that nurses document only interventions that are performed.
- EMR entries cannot be altered or obliterated.
- Use of EHRs can:
  - Reduce storage space
  - Allow simultaneous access by multiple users
  - Facilitate easy duplication for sharing or backup
  - Decrease medication errors
  - Increase portability in environments using wireless systems and handheld devices
  - Enable data retrieval
  - Show trends, for example, of a patient's laboratory work or vital signs

PAPER CHARTING

- Paper medical records are now rarely used except in cases of EHR downtime due to power outages or mass disaster.
- Nurses are still responsible during such time to document accurately.
- Documentation must be completed in ink.
- Do not erase or use correction tape; cross out errors with a single line and initial.
- Date, time, signature, and credentials are required with each entry.
- No blank spaces are left between entries.
- Problems associated with paper charting:
  - Records are available to only one caregiver at a time.
  - Paper is fragile and can degrade over time.
  - Handwriting may be illegible.
  - Storage space is a problem.

HANDOFF REPORTING
Handoff Reporting

- Handoff reporting is passing patient-specific information from one caregiver to another.
- Handoff reports may be oral, in person, or on the phone, or written on the EHR.
- Reports may take place between shifts, between caregivers, or when transferring a patient.
- Handoff reporting should be accurate, timely, essential information.
- Information shared during handoff should support care delivery and clinical decision making.
- During handoff, interprofessional collaboration can occur.
- A consistent handoff process should be used by all caregivers.
- One consistent method of handoff reporting is use of SBAR.

SBAR Reporting

Element	Description
Situation	What is happening at the current time?
Background	What are the circumstances leading up to this situation?
Assessment	What does the nurse think the problem is?
Recommendation	What should we do to correct the problem?

Reprinted from www.IHI.org with permission of the Institute for Healthcare Improvement, © 2019. Retrieved from www.ihi.org/knowledge/pages/tools/sbartoolkit.aspx.

HIPAA

- The Health Insurance Portability and Accountability Act (HIPAA) originally passed in 1996.
- It created standards for the protection of personal health information.
- Patient information is shared only with those who have a need to know.
- EHRs allow sharing of data among caregivers with built-in security.
- Access to an EHR is controlled through passwords and verification codes.
- Never share individual passwords with anyone.
- Ensure that computer screens are not visible to others when in use.
- Log out of the medical record when finished documenting.

SOCIAL MEDIA

- Nurses should follow HIPAA guidelines when using social media.
- Sharing patient information or photos on social media is a violation of HIPAA.
- Be aware that each facility has policies that govern use of social media and other websites on work computers.
- A video, *Social Guidelines Media for Nurses,* is available on the National Council of State Boards of Nursing website at https://www.ncsbn.org/347.htm.
- The American Nurses Association's *Principles for Social Networking and the Nurse* (2011) provides guidelines and assists nurses in understanding the consequences associated with violating online boundary issues.

For additional information on documentation, consult the following:

American Nurses Association (ANA): *Principles for social networking and the nurse.* Silver Springs, Md., 2011, Author.

Balzer Riley J: *Communication in Nursing,* ed 8, St. Louis, 2017, Elsevier.

Potter PA, Perry AG, Stockert PA, Hall AM: *Fundamentals of nursing,* ed 10, St. Louis, 2021, Elsevier.

Yoost BL, Crawford LR: *Conceptual care mapping: case studies for improving communication, collaboration, and care,* St. Louis, 2018, Elsevier.

Yoost BL, Crawford LR: *Fundamentals of nursing: active learning for collaborative practice,* ed 2, St. Louis, 2020, Elsevier.

CHAPTER 6

Patient Interview

FRAMEWORK FOR COLLECTING HEALTH HISTORY DATA

- **Demographic data:** Name, address, telephone numbers, stated age, birth date, birthplace, gender identity, sexual orientation, marital status, race, cultural background or ethnic origin, spiritual or religious preference, educational level, occupation.
- **Chief complaint or present illness:** Reason for seeking care, onset of symptoms.
- **Allergies and sensitivities:** Medication, food (e.g., peanuts, eggs), environmental agents (e.g., latex, tape, detergents), reaction to reported allergens (e.g., rash, breathing difficulty, nausea and vomiting).
- **Medications, vitamins, and herbal supplements:** Prescriptions; over-the-counter medications and herbal remedies; dosage, frequency, and reason for use, including as-needed (PRN) medications.

- **Immunizations:** Childhood and adult immunizations, date of last tuberculin skin test, date of last vaccines (e.g., flu, pneumonia, shingles).
- **Medical history:** Childhood illnesses, accidents, and injuries; serious or chronic illnesses; hospitalizations, including obstetric history for female patients; dates of occurrence; present treatments.
- **Surgical history:** Type of surgery, date, any complications.
- **Family history:** Age and health status of parents, grandparents, siblings, and children; age and cause of death of immediate family members; genetic diseases or traits, familial diseases (e.g., cardiovascular disease, high blood pressure, stroke, blood disorders, cancer, diabetes, kidney disease, seizure disorders, drug or alcohol dependencies, mental illness).
- **Social history:** Caffeine intake; use of tobacco, alcohol, or recreational drugs; environmental exposures; animal exposures and pets; living arrangements; safety concerns (e.g., intimate partner violence, emotional or physical abuse, recent domestic or foreign travel).
- **Cultural and spiritual or religious traditions:** Primary language, dietary restrictions, values and beliefs related to health care.
- **Activities of daily living (ADLs):** Nutrition (e.g., meal preparation, shopping, typical 24-hour dietary intake), any recent changes in appetite, self-care activities (e.g., bathing, dressing, grooming, ambulation), use of prosthetics or mobility devices, leisure and exercise activities, sleep patterns (e.g., hours per night, naps, sleep aids).

- **Cognitive and emotional status:** Cognitive functioning (long-term and short-term memory), personal strengths, self-esteem, support systems (e.g., family, friends, support groups, professional counseling).

GENERAL HEALTH INFORMATION ASSESSMENT QUESTIONS

- How are you feeling?
- What current concerns do you have about your health?
- Do you have any ongoing illnesses?
- Are you in pain? If so, where is the pain located? On a scale of 0 to 10 with 10 being the most severe pain, how do you rate your pain? Describe the pain. How long have you had the pain? Does it radiate anywhere? What relieves the pain or makes it worse?
- Have you ever been hospitalized or had surgery? If so, for what, when, and where?
- Are you up-to-date on your immunizations?
- Are you pregnant or breastfeeding?
- Describe your energy level. Are you able to participate in your daily activities without being fatigued or short of breath?
- Describe any significant life stresses you are experiencing. Do you feel safe at home?

MEDICATION/VITAMIN/HERBAL SUPPLEMENT ASSESSMENT QUESTIONS

Drug History and Current Use

- What food or drug allergies do you have? Describe the reaction.
- What prescribed medications are you currently taking? Dosage and frequency? Do you have them with you?

- Which over-the-counter medications, vitamins, and herbal supplements do you take on a regular basis (e.g., antacids, laxatives, aspirin, creams, or lotions)? Dosage and frequency?
- How many alcoholic beverages do you consume each day? How many caffeinated beverages each day?
- What medications have you stopped taking recently?
- Do you use any other methods to relieve your symptoms? What home remedies have you tried?
- Do you have any cultural or religious considerations regarding medications?

Medication Schedule
- What times do you take your medications?
- Do you prepare your medications in a special way (e.g., crushed in applesauce, taken with a meal)?
- How do you remember to take your medications on schedule?

Medication Response
- What response have you had to your medications?
- Have you had any side effects or adverse reactions from medications?

Medication Compliance
- Can you tell me why you take this medication?
- Are there problems that prevent you from taking your medications (e.g., cost, access at work or school, irregular meal schedules)?
- Do you have vision problems? Hearing problems? Difficulty opening medication containers? Mobility difficulties? Trouble remembering to take medications? Trouble swallowing?
- How do you feel about taking medications?

Medication Safety
- Where are your medications kept at home?
- Do others have access to your medications? Any children or teens?
- Do you have medications at home that you no longer take regularly? How long do you keep your medications?
- How do you dispose of medications that you are no longer taking?
- Do you do any special monitoring for these medications (e.g., blood levels, blood glucose monitoring)?

CULTURAL ASSESSMENT QUESTIONS
(Adapt according to specific patient needs.)

Communication
- What do you do to help others understand what you are trying to say?
- Do you like communicating with friends, family members, and acquaintances?
- When asked a question, do you usually respond in words, body movement, or both?
- If you have something important to discuss with your family, how do you approach them?

Space
- When you talk with family members, how close do you stand?
- When you communicate with coworkers and others, how close do you stand?
- If a stranger touches you, how do you react or feel?
- If a loved one touches you, how do you react or feel?
- Are you comfortable with the distance between us now?

Social Organization

- How do you define social activities?
- What are some activities that you enjoy?
- What are your hobbies? What do you do in your free time?
- What is your role in the family unit?
- What is your function in the family unit?
- When you were younger, who influenced you the most?
- What does work mean to you?
- Describe your past, present, and future jobs.

Time

- What methods do you use to keep track of time each day?
- If you have an appointment at 2 p.m., what is an acceptable arrival time?
- If the nurse tells you that you will receive a medication in "about half an hour," realistically, how much time will you allow before you call the nurses' station about the medication?

Environmental Control

- How often do you have visitors to your home?
- Is it acceptable to you for visitors to drop in unannounced?
- What is your definition of good health?
- What is your definition of poor health?
- What home remedies have you used that worked?
- Will you use these home remedies again?

Biologic Variations

- What illnesses or diseases are common in your family?
- Have any members of your family been told they have a genetic susceptibility to a particular disease?

- How do you respond when you are angry?
- Who or what helps you cope during difficult times?
- What foods do you and your family like?
- Have you ever had any cravings for unusual things such as red or white clay? Laundry starch?
- What foods are family favorites or traditional foods?

Adapted from Giger J: *Transcultural nursing: Assessment and intervention,* ed 7, St. Louis, 2017, Elsevier.

SPIRITUAL ASSESSMENT QUESTIONS

- Do you have family in the area? (Assess for family importance, relationships, and meaningful experiences at this time.)
- Is there anyone you would like to call?
- How are you handling this hospitalization or illness?
- What faith practices or beliefs will help you cope with this illness or hospitalization?
- Do you have any dietary or treatment guidelines/restrictions related to your spiritual/religious beliefs?
- Do you belong to a faith community? Do you want the community to be notified? Would you like a chaplain to visit?

SLEEP ASSESSMENT QUESTIONS

- How have you been sleeping?
- Do you have any bedtime routines?
- What time do you usually go to bed?
- What time do you usually awaken?
- Do you feel rested when you awaken?

- How long does it take for you to go to sleep?
- Do you awaken during the night? How often? What do you do?
- Do you have enough energy to complete your tasks during the day?
- Do you take naps during the day? For how long?
- What is your normal eating pattern?
- Do you drink beverages with caffeine, such as colas, coffee, or tea?
- Does your sleep partner comment about your sleep? Snoring? Pauses in breathing?
- What do you do to help yourself sleep? Use of over-the-counter meds? Prescription meds?

SEXUALITY ASSESSMENT QUESTIONS

- How do you feel about the sexual aspect of your life?
- Have you noticed any changes in the way you see yourself (as a man, woman, husband, wife, partner)?
- How has your illness, surgery, or medication affected your sex life?
- Are you active sexually?
- Do you have problems or concerns regarding your sexual abilities, performance, or satisfaction?
- How many sexual partners have you had in your lifetime?
- What are or have been your sexual practices?
- Do you feel safe in your environment?

    From Yoost BL, Crawford LR: *Fundamentals of nursing: active learning for collaborative practice*, ed 2, St. Louis, 2020, Elsevier.

For additional information on interviewing patients,
consult the following:

Giger J: *Transcultural nursing: Assessment and intervention,* ed 7, St. Louis, 2017, Mosby.

Potter PA, Perry AG, Stockert PA, Hall AM: *Fundamentals of nursing,* ed 10, St. Louis, 2021, Elsevier.

Yoost BL, Crawford LR: *Fundamentals of nursing: active learning for collaborative practice,* ed 2, St. Louis, 2020, Elsevier.

Yoost BL, Crawford LR: *Conceptual Care Mapping: case studies for improving communication, collaboration, and care,* St. Louis, 2018, Elsevier.

CHAPTER 7

Vital Signs

SITUATIONS THAT REQUIRE VITAL SIGN ASSESSMENT

- Establishing a baseline on admission to a health care agency.
- As part of a physical assessment.
- Routine monitoring during an inpatient stay.
- With any change in health status, especially complaints of chest pain and shortness of breath or feeling hot, faint, or dizzy.
- Before and after surgery or invasive procedures to establish baselines and monitor effects.
- Before and after administration of medications that affect cardiac, respiratory, or thermal regulation systems.
- Before and after interventions such as ambulation.
- Detecting improvement in patient condition.
- Validating readiness for discharge or transfer from a unit.
- Before and after a medication that affects cardiovascular and respiratory function.

VITAL SIGN RANGES ACROSS THE LIFE SPAN

Age Group	Temperature	Pulse (bpm)	Respirations (bpm)	SpO₂	Blood Pressure (mm Hg)	
					Systolic	Diastolic
Newborn	35.5°-37.5°C (96°-99.5°F)	80-160	30-80	>95%	60-90	20-60
1 yr old	37.4°-37.6°C (99.4°-99.7°F)	80-140	24-40	>95%	74-100	50-70
6 yr old	36.6°-37°C (98°-98.6°F)	75-110	15-25	>95%	84-<120	54-<80
15 yr old	36.1°-37.2°C (97°-99°F)	50-90	15-20	>95%	94-<120	62-<80
Adult	35.5°-37.5°C (95.9°-99.5°F)	60-100	12-20	>95%	90-<120	60-<80
Older adult	35°-37.2°C (95°-99°F)	60-100	15-20	>95%	90-<120	60-<80

From Yoost BL, Crawford LR: *Fundamentals of nursing: active learning for collaborative practice,* ed 2, St. Louis, 2020, Elsevier.

TEMPERATURE
Clinical Signs of Fever
Onset: Increased heart rate, increased respirations, pallor, cool skin, cyanosis, chills, decreased sweating, and increased temperature.

Course: Flushed, warm skin; increased heart rate and respiration; increased thirst; mild dehydration; drowsiness; restlessness; decreased appetite; weakness.

Reduction: Flushed skin, decreased shivering, dehydration, diaphoresis.

Average Adult Temperature Ranges at Different Body Sites

Assessment Method	Fahrenheit	Centigrade
Oral	96.8°-99.68°	36.0°-37.6°
Axillary	95.9°-98.6°	35.5°-37.0°
Rectal	93.92°-100.04°	34.4°-37.8°
Tympanic	96.08°-99.32°	35.6°-37.4°
Temporal	96.98°-99.14°	36.1°-37.3°

From Yoost BL, Crawford LR: *Fundamentals of nursing: active learning for collaborative practice,* ed 2, St. Louis, 2020, Elsevier.

Factors Affecting Temperature
Age: Infants and elderly adults respond drastically to change in temperature.

Exercise: Increasing exercise will increase heat production and increase body temperature.

Hormones: Fluctuations in hormones can cause fluctuations in temperature.

Stress: Physical and emotional stress can increase body temperature.

Circadian rhythm: Lower temperatures in morning; higher in afternoon and evening.

Temperature-Related Disorders
Hypothermia
Stage 1: Body temperature drops by 1°C to 2°C (1.8°F to 3.6°F). Shivering occurs. Unable to perform complex tasks with the hands. Blood vessels in the outer extremities contract. Breathing becomes quick and shallow. Goose bumps form to create an insulating layer of air around the body.
Treatment: Warm slowly.
Stage 2: Body temperature drops by 2°C to 4°C (3.6°F to 7.2°F). Shivering becomes violent. Muscle discoordination becomes apparent. Mild confusion, although the victim may appear alert. Victim becomes pale, and lips, ears, fingers, and toes may be blue.
Treatment: Warm slowly.
Stage 3: Body temperature drops below approximately 32°C or 90°F. Shivering may stop, and difficulty speaking, sluggish thinking, and amnesia appear; inability to use hands and stumbling are usually present. Skin becomes blue and puffy, muscle coordination very poor, walking nearly impossible, and the victim exhibits incoherent or irrational behavior. Pulse and respiration rates decrease, but ventricular tachycardia or atrial fibrillation can occur. Major organs fail.
Treatment: Warm slowly.
Frostbite: Damage to skin caused by extreme cold. At or below 0°C (32°F), blood vessels close to the skin constrict.
Treatment: Warm slowly.
Heatstroke: Temperature above 42.2°C or 108°F.
Treatment: Ice to groin and axilla.
Heat cramps: Spasms of muscles.
Treatment: Replace fluids; watch for chilling.

Hyperthermia: Any temperature above normal; severe hyperthermia is indicated by temperatures at or above 42.2°C or 108°F.

Treatment: Replace fluids; watch for chilling.

PULSE

Average Adult Pulse Rate Range
60–100 beats per minute

Rhythm
- The pulse rhythm is typically regular. An irregular rhythm in the pulse is caused by an early, late, or missed heartbeat.
- An irregular pulse rhythm is referred to as a dysrhythmia or an arrhythmia.

Pulse Deficit
- A pulse deficit is present when the patient's radial pulse rate is slower than the apical pulse rate because of cardiac contractions that are weak or ineffective at pumping blood to the peripheral tissues and extremities.

Apical Pulse Assessment
- The apical pulse is auscultated with a stethoscope for a full minute at the apex of the heart on the anterior chest wall.
- It is best heard between the left fifth and sixth intercostal spaces over the midclavicular line.

Peripheral Pulse Intensity
0 = Absent
1 = Weaker than expected or thready; may be difficult to palpate
2 = Normal; able to palpate with normal pressure
3 = Bounding; may be able to see pulsation; doesn't disappear with palpation

Factors Affecting Pulse Rate

Age: As age increases from infancy to adulthood, the pulse rate decreases.

Gender: After puberty, the average male pulse is lower than that of the average female.

Fever: Pulse increases with fever due to the increased metabolic rate and peripheral vasodilation that occurs.

Pain: Pain will increase the rate of a person's pulse.

Stress: Sympathetic nervous system stimulation from stress (e.g., fear, anxiety, and the perception of pain) increases the heart rate.

Digestion: The increased metabolic rate during digestion will increase the pulse rate.

Medications: Medications may either increase or decrease the pulse rate.

Hypovolemia: Loss of blood will typically increase the pulse rate from sympathetic nervous system stimulation.

Hypoxia and hypoxemia: When oxygen levels decrease, cardiac output increases to attempt to compensate, resulting in an increased pulse rate.

Blood pressure: In general, heart rate and blood pressure have an inverse relationship. When the blood pressure is low, there is an increase in pulse rate as the heart attempts to increase its output of blood (cardiac output).

Electrolyte balance: Changes in potassium and calcium affect pulse rate and rhythm.

Pulse Sites

- **Temporal***: Where the temporal artery passes over the temporal bone of the head, above and lateral to the eye; used when the radial pulse is not accessible.
- **Carotid***: At the side of the neck where the carotid artery runs between the trachea and the

sternocleidomastoid muscle; used in cases of cardiac arrest and for determining circulation to the brain.

- **Apical or PMI:** Apical, at the apex of the heart, and PMI, at the fifth intercostal space, midclavicular line; used for infants and children up to 3 years of age, placed in the supine position, to determine discrepancies with radial pulse, and used in adults in conjunction with some diseases and medications and during a head-to-toe assessment.
- **Brachial:** At the inner aspect of the arm; used to assess pulse in pediatric emergencies and to measure blood pressure.
- **Radial*:** On the thumb side of the inner aspect of the wrist where the radial artery runs along the radial bone.
- **Femoral:** Where the femoral artery passes alongside the inguinal ligament; used in cases of cardiac arrest and for assessing circulation to the leg.
- **Popliteal:** Behind the knee where the popliteal artery passes; used to determine circulation to the lower leg.
- **Posterior tibial:** Medial surface of the ankle; used to determine circulation to the foot.
- **Dorsalis pedis:** Where the dorsalis pedis artery passes across the top of the foot; used to determine circulation to the foot.

---

*The radial pulse typically is readily accessible. In elderly people, however, palpating the radial pulse may pose a challenge if tremors are present. Peripheral pulses also may be decreased in general because of cardiovascular changes with aging.

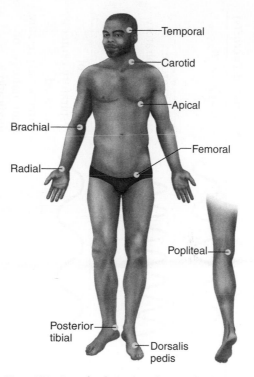

(From Yoost BL, Crawford LR: *Fundamentals of nursing: active learning for collaborative practice*, ed 2, St. Louis, 2020, Elsevier.)

RESPIRATION
Average Adult Respiratory Rate Range
12–20 breaths per minute

Respiratory Patterns Including Depth and Quality

Pattern	Description		Associated Factor(s)
Eupnea	Quiet, regular breathing; 12-20 bpm	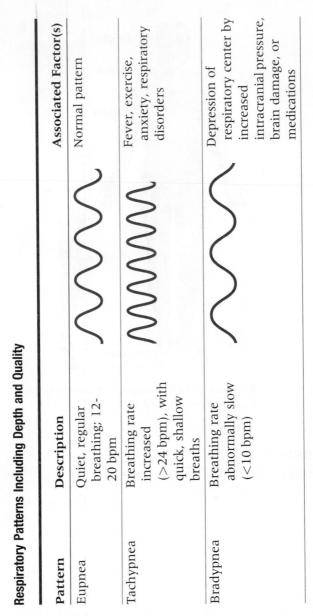	Normal pattern
Tachypnea	Breathing rate increased (>24 bpm), with quick, shallow breaths		Fever, exercise, anxiety, respiratory disorders
Bradypnea	Breathing rate abnormally slow (<10 bpm)		Depression of respiratory center by increased intracranial pressure, brain damage, or medications

Respiratory Patterns Including Depth and Quality—Cont'd

Pattern	Description		Associated Factor(s)
Hyperventilation	Overexpansion of the lungs, characterized by rapid and deep breaths		Extreme exercise, fear, anxiety, diabetic ketoacidosis, aspirin overdose
Hypoventilation	Underexpansion of the lungs, characterized by shallow, slow respirations		Drug overdose, head injury
Cheyne-Stokes respirations	Rhythmic respirations, going from very deep to very shallow or apneic periods		Heart failure, renal failure, drug overdose, increased intracranial pressure, impending death

Continued

Respiratory Patterns Including Depth and Quality—Cont'd

Pattern	Description		Associated Factor(s)
Kussmaul's breathing	Respirations abnormally deep, regular, and increased in rate		Diabetic ketoacidosis
Apnea	Absence of breathing for several seconds		Respiratory distress, obstructive sleep apnea
Biot's breathing	Respirations abnormally shallow for two or three breaths, followed by irregular period of apnea		Meningitis, severe brain injury

From Yoost BL, Crawford LR: *Fundamentals of nursing: active learning for collaborative practice*, ed 2, St. Louis, 2020, Elsevier.

Adventitious Breath Sounds

- **Crackles:** Most often in the lung bases and position-dependent lobes. Caused by the sudden opening of small airways and alveoli collapsed by fluid, exudate, or lack of air flow during expiration, pneumonia, atelectasis, cystic fibrosis, bronchitis, or pulmonary edema.
- **Pleural friction rub:** Low-pitched, grating, or creaking sound. Can be described as the sound made by treading on fresh snow. Present over anterior lateral thorax, midline to axillae. Present during inspiration or expiration and is not cleared by cough. Occurs when inflamed pleural surfaces rub together during respiration.
- **Rhonchi:** Low-pitched, snore-like sounds heard either during inspiration or expiration, usually clear with a cough. Continuous sounds, mainly heard over trachea and bronchi. Almost always caused by increased secretions in large airways.
- **Stridor:** Intense, high-pitched, and continuous. Heard during inspiration, often heard without the aid of a stethoscope. Heard over trachea and large airways. Most often caused by epiglottitis, a foreign body lodged in the airway, or a laryngeal tumor.
- **Wheezing:** High-pitched, whistling sound, heard continuously during inspiration or expiration; most obvious and loudest during exhalation.

Factors Affecting Respiratory Rate and Depth

Age: Respiratory rate decreases with age through late adolescence, when it stabilizes.

Exercise: Respiratory rate and depth increase with exercise.

Illness processes: Cardiovascular disease and hematologic disorders such as anemia cause an increased respiratory rate. Sickle cell disease reduces the ability of hemoglobin to carry oxygen, resulting in increased respiratory rate and depth.

Respiratory diseases can be manifested by difficulty breathing, use of accessory muscles, increased rate, and more shallow depth. Smoking alters airways, resulting in an increased rate.

Acid–base balance: Acidosis results in increased rate and depth of respirations in an attempt to rid the body of excess carbon dioxide. Alkalosis results in decreased respiratory rate as the body tries to retain carbon dioxide.

Medications: Some medications, such as narcotics and general anesthesia, slow respirations. Alternatively, drugs such as amphetamines and cocaine increase respirations. Bronchodilators slow the respiratory rate by dilating the airways.

Pain: Acute pain increases respiratory rate while decreasing respiratory depth.

Emotions: Fear or anxiety can cause increased respiratory rate and decreased depth.

OXYGEN SATURATION
Normal Range of Oxygen Saturation (SpO$_2$)
95% to 100%

Factors that affect Oxygen Saturation
- Lung disease
- Decreased circulation
- Hypotension

BLOOD PRESSURE
Categories for Blood Pressure Levels in Adults*

Category	Systolic (mm Hg)		Diastolic (mm Hg)
Hypotension	<90	*or*	<60
Normal	<120	*and*	<80

Continued

Categories for Blood Pressure Levels in Adults—Cont'd

Category	Systolic (mm Hg)		Diastolic (mm Hg)
Elevated	120-129	*and*	<80
Hypertension stage 1	130-139	*or*	80–89
Hypertension stage 2	≥140	*or*	≥90

*People 18 years of age and older who are not on medications for high blood pressure or other conditions that affect blood pressure.

From Yoost BL, Crawford LR: *Fundamentals of nursing: active learning for collaborative practice,* ed 2, St. Louis, 2020, Elsevier.

Korotkoff Sounds

Phase	Description
Korotkoff I	The initial presentation of faint but clearly audible tapping sounds, which gradually increase in intensity to a thud or loud tap; the first sound is recorded as the systolic pressure
Korotkoff II	Muffled, swishing sounds
Korotkoff III	Crisp, loud sounds as the blood flows through an opening artery
Korotkoff IV	A distinct, abrupt muffling sound
Korotkoff V	The last sound heard before silence—this is the diastolic measurement

From Yoost BL, Crawford LR: *Fundamentals of nursing: active learning for collaborative practice,* ed 2, St. Louis, 2020, Elsevier.

Blood Pressure Cuff Sizing

Blood pressure cuff should be approximately 60% to 80% of the circumference of the extremity being used, and the width of the cuff should be approximately 40% of the circumference of the extremity.

Causes of False Blood Pressure Readings

False High Reading
- Having a cuff that is too narrow
- Having a cuff that is too short
- Deflating the cuff too slowly
- Having the arm below the heart
- Having the arm unsupported
- Assessing blood pressure too soon after patient smoking or exercise
- Releasing the pressure valve too slowly
- Reinflating the bladder before it has completely deflated

False Low Reading
- Having a cuff that is too wide
- Having a cuff that is too long
- Deflating the cuff too quickly
- Having the arm above the heart
- Hearing deficit of assessing person
- Ear tips of stethoscope placed incorrectly
- Breaks or kinks in cuff tubing
- Not placing stethoscope bell directly over artery

False Diastolic Reading
- Deflating the cuff too slowly
- Having a stethoscope that fits poorly in the examiner's ears
- Inflating the cuff too slowly

False Systolic Reading
- Deflating the cuff too quickly
  From Potter PA, Perry AG, Stockert PA, Hall AM: *Fundamentals of nursing,* ed 9, St. Louis, 2017, Elsevier.

Orthostatic Hypotension

- Measured by taking the blood pressure reading and pulse while the patient is in the lying position, sitting position, and standing position.
- Orthostatic hypotension is present when a patient changes from supine to a sitting or standing position if there is:
  - A drop in blood pressure of 20 mm Hg systolic or 10 mm Hg diastolic, or
  - An increase in heart rate of 20 bpm

For additional information on vital sign assessment, consult the following:

Ball JW, et al: *Seidel's guide to physical examination,* ed 9, St. Louis, 2019, Elsevier

Jarvis C: *Physical examination and health assessment,* ed 8, St. Louis, 2020, Elsevier.

Potter PA, Perry AG, Stockert PA, Hall AM: *Fundamentals of nursing,* ed 10, St. Louis, 2021, Elsevier.

Wilson SF, Giddens JF: *Health assessment for nursing practice,* ed 6, St. Louis, 2017, Elsevier

Yoost BL, Crawford LR: *Fundamentals of nursing: active learning for collaborative practice,* ed 2, St. Louis, 2020, Elsevier.

CHAPTER 8

Physical Assessment

General Survey (p. 90)
Assessment Techniques (p. 91)

GENERAL SURVEY

Appearance
Stage of development, general health, striking features, height, weight, behavior, posture, communication skills, grooming, hygiene

Skin
Color, consistency, temperature, turgor, integrity, texture, lesions, mucous membranes

Hair
Color, texture, amount, distribution

Nails
Color, texture, shape, size

Neurologic
Pupil reaction, motor and verbal responses, gait, reflexes, neurologic checks

Musculoskeletal
Range of motion, gait, tone, posture

Cardiovascular
Heart rate and rhythm, peripheral pulses and temperature, edema

Respiratory
Rate, rhythm, depth, effort, quality, expansion, cough, breath sounds, sputum (production, color, and amount), tracheostomy presence and size, nasal patency

Gastrointestinal
Abdominal contour, bowel sounds, nausea, vomiting, ostomy type and care, fecal frequency, consistency, presence of blood

Genitourinary
Urine color, character, amount, odor, ostomy type and care

ASSESSMENT TECHNIQUES
- The assessment techniques of inspection, palpation, percussion, and auscultation are performed one at a time in that order for each body system except during assessment of the abdomen.
- During abdominal assessment, auscultation precedes palpation and percussion.*

Inspection: Use of vision, hearing, and smell to closely scrutinize physical characteristics of a whole person and individual body systems. Symmetry should be assessed by comparing the right and left sides of the body.

Palpation: Use of touch to assess body organs and skin texture, temperature, moisture, turgor, tenderness, and thickness. Palpation can determine organ location and size against the expected anatomic norm, any distention or masses, and vibration or pulsation associated with movement. Only light palpation should be applied to areas described by patients as sensitive or painful.

---

*If assessing the abdomen, auscultate before palpation and percussion.

Light Palpation

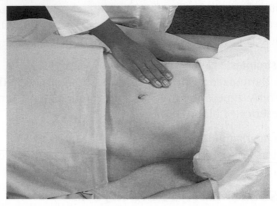

Light palpation of the abdomen. With fingers extended and approximated, press in no more than 1 cm. (From Ball JW, et al.: *Seidel's guide to physical examination,* ed 9, St. Louis, 2019, Elsevier.)

Deep Palpation

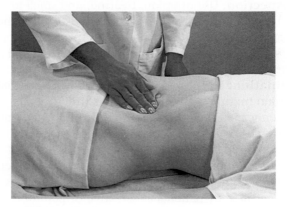

Deep single hand palpation.

Continued

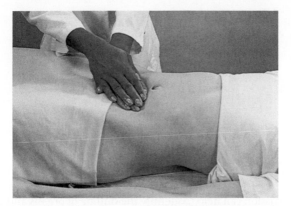

Deep bimanual palpation. (From Ball JW, et al.: *Seidel's guide to physical examination,* ed 9, St. Louis, 2019, Elsevier.)

Percussion: Tapping the patient's skin with short, sharp strokes that cause a vibration to travel through the skin and to the upper layers of the underlying structures. Vibration is reflected by the tissues, and the character of the sound heard depends on the density of the structures that reflect the sound. Knowing how the various densities reflect or absorb sound helps to determine the approximate size, shape, and borders of organs, masses, and fluid. Percussion is an advanced practice examination technique.

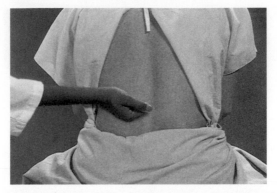

Percussion can help to identify the outline of organs and the possible presence of masses. (From Ball JW, et al.: *Seidel's guide to physical examination,* ed 9, St. Louis, 2019, Elsevier.)

Auscultation: Listening with the assistance of a stethoscope to sounds made by organs or systems such as the heart, blood vessels, lungs, and abdominal cavity. The characteristics of auscultated sounds depend on the body tissue or organ being assessed. Breath sounds, heart sounds, and bowel sounds are routinely assessed through auscultation.

• Remember that auscultation precedes palpation and percussion during abdominal assessment.

For additional information on physical assessment, consult the following:

Ball JW, et al: *Seidel's guide to physical examination,* ed 9, St. Louis, 2019, Elsevier.

Jarvis C: *Physical examination and health assessment,* ed 8, St. Louis, 2020, Elsevier.

Potter PA, Perry AG, Stockert PA, Hall AM: *Fundamentals of nursing,* ed 10, St. Louis, 2021, Elsevier.

Wilson SF, Giddens JF: *Health assessment for nursing practice,* ed 6, St. Louis, 2017, Elsevier.

Yoost BL, Crawford LR: *Fundamentals of nursing: active learning for collaborative practice,* ed 2, St. Louis, 2020, Elsevier.

CHAPTER 9

Pain Assessment

PAIN ASSESSMENT QUESTIONS

- What is the intensity of your pain? Would you describe your pain as mild, moderate, or severe? On a pain scale with 0 being no pain and 10 being excruciating pain, how do you rate your pain?
- How long have you been experiencing this pain? Has the pain begun recently, or have you been in pain longer than 6 months?
- Where is the pain you are experiencing? Does it radiate anywhere? Point to exactly where the pain is and where it radiates to, if it does.
- Have you noticed any pattern with the pain you are experiencing? Does the pain occur in the morning, occur when you are ambulating, or awaken you during the night?
- Is the pain sharp or dull, aching or throbbing, or burning? Is the pain constant or intermittent (comes and goes)?
- Are there precipitating factors that occur before the pain is felt? What have you tried for pain relief? Have you tried applying heat or ice packs, or massaging or rubbing the area? Has anything you have tried helped?
- What medications are you currently using or have you taken in the past to relieve pain?

UNIVERSAL PAIN ASSESSMENT TOOL

This pain assessment tool is intended to help patient care providers assess pain according to individual patient needs. Explain and use and use 0 to 10 Scale for patient self assessment. Use the faces or behavioral observations to interpret expressed pain when patient cannot communicate his or her pain intensity.

0 to 10 Scale	0	1	2	3	4	5	6	7	8	9	10
Verbal Descriptor Scale	NO PAIN		MILD PAIN		MODERATE PAIN		MODERATE PAIN		SEVERE PAIN		WORST PAIN POSSIBLE
Wong-Baker FACES Pain Rating Scale	NO HURT		HURTS LITTLE BIT		HURTS LITTLE MORE		HURTS EVEN MORE		HURTS WHOLE LOT		HURTS WORST
Activity Tolerance Scale	NO PAIN		CAN BE IGNORED		INTERFERES WITH TASKS		INTERFERES WITH CONCENTRATION		INTERFERES WITH BASIC NEEDS		BEDREST REQUIRED

Visual cues, descriptive terms, and activity levels can be useful in helping patients identify their level of pain if they are unable to relate to the numeric scale. (From Wong-Baker FACES Foundation (2018). Wong-Baker FACES Pain Rating Scale. Retrieved with permission from http://www.WongBakerFACES.org.

PAIN ASSESSMENT MNEMONICS

SOCRATES

- **S**: Site (Where is the pain located?)
- **O**: Onset (When did the pain start? Was it gradual or sudden?)
- **C**: Character (What is the quality of the pain? Is it stabbing, burning, or aching?)
- **R**: Radiation (Does the pain radiate anywhere?)
- **A**: Associations (What signs and symptoms are associated with the pain?)
- **T**: Time course (Is there a pattern to when the pain occurs?)
- **E**: Exacerbating or relieving factors (Does anything make the pain worse or lessen it?)
- **S**: Severity (On a scale of 0 to 10, what is the intensity of the pain?)

PQRST

- **P**: Provocation (initiating factor)
- **Q**: Quality
- **R**: Region (location)
- **S**: Severity
- **T**: Temporality (onset, duration, fluctuation)

OLDCARTS

- **O**: Onset
- **L**: Location/radiation
- **D**: Duration
- **C**: Character
- **A**: Aggravating factors
- **R**: Relieving factors
- **T**: Timing
- **S**: Severity

CLINICAL MANIFESTATIONS OF PAIN

Body system	Clinical manifestations
Cardiovascular	Increased heart rate and force of contraction in acute pain
	Increased systolic blood pressure in acute pain
	Decreased systolic blood pressure in prolonged pain or chronic pain
	Decreased pulse in prolonged pain or chronic pain
	Increased myocardial oxygen demand
	Increased vascular resistance
	Hypercoagulation
	Chest pain
Respiratory	Increased respiratory rate
	Increased bronchospasms
	Pneumonia
	Atelectasis
Gastrointestinal	Delayed gastric emptying
	Decreased intestinal motility
	Constipation
	Anorexia
	Weight loss
Musculoskeletal	Muscle spasms
	Increased muscle tension
	Impaired mobility
	Weakness
	Fatigue
Endocrine	Fever
	Shock

CLINICAL MANIFESTATIONS
OF PAIN—Cont'd

Body system	Clinical manifestations
Genitourinary	Decreased urine output Urinary retention Fluid overload Hypokalemia
Sensory	Pallor Diaphoresis Dilated pupils in acute pain Constricted pupils in deep or prolonged pain Rapid speech in acute pain Slow speech in deep or prolonged pain
Immune	Impaired immune function Infection

From Yoost BL, Crawford LR: *Fundamentals of nursing: active learning for collaborative practice,* ed 2, St. Louis, 2020, Elsevier.

TIMING OF PAIN ASSESSMENT AFTER TREATMENT

Nonpharmacologic techniques	30-60 min after intervention
Intramuscular (IM), subcutaneous (subcut), or oral (PO) administration	30-60 min after intervention
Transdermal administration	12-16 hr after intervention
Intravenous (IV) or sublingual administration	15-30 min after intervention

For additional information on pain assessment,
consult the following:

Ball JW, et al: *Seidel's guide to physical examination,* ed 9, St. Louis, 2019, Elsevier.

Jarvis C: *Physical examination and health assessment*, ed 8, St. Louis, 2020, Elsevier.

Potter PA, Perry AG, Stockert PA, Hall AM: *Fundamentals of nursing*, ed 10, St. Louis, 2021, Elsevier.

Wilson SF, Giddens JF: *Health assessment for nursing practice,* ed 6, St. Louis, 2017, Elsevier.

Yoost BL, Crawford LR: *Fundamentals of nursing: active learning for collaborative practice*, ed 2, St. Louis, 2020, Elsevier.

CHAPTER 10

Skin, Hair, and Nail Assessment

SKIN, HAIR, AND NAIL HEALTH ASSESSMENT QUESTIONS

- Have you observed any noticeable changes in the consistency, color, or texture of your skin, hair, or nails recently? Is your skin normally dry, oily, or a combination of both?
- Has anyone in your family ever had skin cancer? Do you have any birthmarks, moles, or tattoos? Have any of them changed in color, size, or shape?
- List any allergic skin reactions you have ever had to food, drugs, plants, or other daily encountered substances.
- Do you have any problems with perspiration, malodorous skin in the absence of perspiration, or itching?
- How much sun or tanning-bed exposure do you have in the average week? What type of sun protection do you use, and how often?
- In your daily activities or occupation, is your skin exposed to chemicals, excessive temperatures, petroleum, bleach, or caustic cleaning products?

- Describe your normal hair texture. How often do you wash your hair? What types of grooming products do you typically use, and how often? Do you ever use chemicals on your hair?
- Have you noticed any generalized hair loss, bald spots, or loss of hair in a specific location? Have you noticed any lumps or painful areas around hair follicles?
- Have you experienced recent changes in your diet or appetite?
- Have you recently undergone chemotherapy or radiation treatment? Are you on any new medications that may cause hair loss or growth?
- Do you have a familial history of male pattern baldness? If so, at what age did it begin?
- Describe any changes you have had in the appearance or condition of your nails.
- Do any skin, hair, or nail problems limit your normal activities?

SKIN INSPECTION AND PALPATION
Color
Cyanosis: Blue discoloration of the skin, nail beds, or mucous membranes that results from vasoconstriction or deoxygenated hemoglobin in blood vessels near the skin's surface.

Erythema: Redness of the skin caused by congestion or dilation of the superficial blood vessels in the skin, signaling circulatory changes to an area. Erythema is not easily detected in dark-skinned people but may be present in an area of the skin that is edematous (swollen) or warmer than the surrounding skin.

Purpura: Bleeding underneath the skin and red pigmentation that does not blanch with pressure are nonspecific signs. Purpura may indicate vascular, coagulation, or platelet disorders.

Jaundice: Yellow hue to the skin, mucous membranes, or eyes seen in both light- and dark-skinned people. The yellow pigment results from excess bilirubin, a byproduct of red blood cell destruction, or liver failure. The best site for evaluation of the patient for jaundice is the sclera or, in darker-skinned people, the hard palate.

Pallor: Pale or lightened skin tone, usually uniformly disseminated throughout the skin surface. Pallor can be caused by illness, emotional shock or stress, decreased exposure to sunlight, or anemia, or may be a genetic trait. It is most easily observed on the face, oral mucosa, nail beds, palms of the hands, and conjunctiva of the eye.

Vitiligo: A loss of skin pigment. It is thought to result from an autoimmune response. Patches of depigmented skin most often are noted on the hands, face, and genital areas.

Turgor: The skin's elasticity or ability to resist deformity after being displaced. Assessed by grasping a fold of skin (1/2 to 1 inch in thickness) on the forearm or over the sternum along the second or third intercostal space and gently pinching the fingertips together and then releasing.

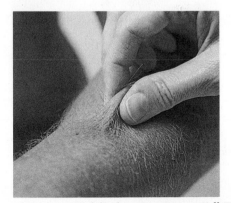

Skin turgor assessment of the forearm. (From Ball JW, et al.: *Seidel's guide to physical examination,* ed 9, St. Louis, 2019, Elsevier.)

Edema: Swelling caused when there is a buildup of fluid in underlying tissues. Common causes of edema are localized trauma to an area and impairment of venous return. Edema secondary to poor venous return usually is most prominent in the lower extremities or dependent areas of the body (e.g., the feet, ankles, and lower legs).

Documentation of Pitting Edema

1+	Slight pitting, 2 mm
2+	Deeper pitting, 4 mm
3+	Deep pitting, 6 mm; dependent extremity enlarged
4+	Very deep pitting, 8 mm; dependent extremity extremely distorted

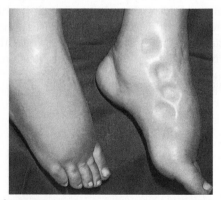

Pitting edema. (From Patton KT, Thibodeau GA: *Anatomy and physiology,* ed. 9, St. Louis, 2016, Elsevier.)

Primary Skin Lesions

Description	Examples	Skin cutaway
Macule/Patch		
Flat, not detectable with palpation Changes in color Size <1 cm >1 cm macule: called a *patch*	Port wine stain Flat moles	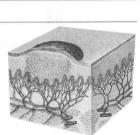
Papule/Plaque		
Solid, raised lesion with distinct borders Variety of shapes: domed, flat-topped, umbilicated Often associated with secondary features: crusts or scales Size <0.5 cm >0.5 cm papule: referred to as a *plaque*	Wart Psoriasis Actinic keratosis	

Continued

Primary Skin Lesions—Cont'd

Description	Examples	Skin cutaway
Nodule		
Raised solid mass with defined borders Extends into the dermis or beyond Deeper and more solid than a papule Size 0.5-2 cm	Lipomas Squamous cell cancers	
Tumor		
Solid mass that extends through subcutaneous tissue May have undefined borders Not always cancerous; may be larger lipomas Nodules that typically are >1-2 cm	Larger lipomas Cancerous lesions	

Primary Skin Lesions—Cont'd

Description	Examples	Skin cutaway
Vesicle/Bulla		
Circumscribed, raised lesions Filled with serous (clear) fluid Size <0.5 cm Vesicles >0.5 cm: referred to as *bullae*	Chickenpox (varicella) Poison ivy Second-degree burn blisters	
Pustule		
Similar to vesicle Circumcised, elevated lesion containing pus instead of clear fluid Most commonly infected	Impetigo Acne	
Wheal		
Irregularly shaped area of edema Caused by serous fluid in the dermis Varies in color and size	Hives (urticaria) Insect bites	

Continued

Primary Skin Lesions—Cont'd

Description	Examples	Skin cutaway
Burrow		
Linear or circular in appearance Caused by infestation and tunneling of parasitic organisms	Scabies mites Ringworms	
Cyst		
Encapsulated fluid-filled or semisolid mass Extends into the dermis or subcutaneous tissue	Sebaceous cyst	

From Yoost BL, Crawford LR: *Fundamentals of nursing: active learning for collaborative practice,* ed 2, St. Louis, 2020, Elsevier.

Pressure Injuries and Braden Scale
See Chapter 24, Wound Care, p. 278.

TYPES OF SKIN CANCER

Description	Risk factors	Symptoms
Basal Cell Carcinoma (BCC)		
Most common skin cancer worldwide Slow growing	Sun exposure Fair complexion Familial history	Bump or scaly growth Does not heal within

TYPES OF SKIN CANCER—Cont'd

Description	Risk factors	Symptoms
Basal Cell Carcinoma (BCC)–Cont'd		
Usually does not metastasize May cause destruction and disfigurement of surrounding tissues	of skin cancer Weakened immune system History of radiation therapy Increased age	2 weeks Begins to itch or bleed May begin at size of 0.5-1 cm and grow Slightly raised or flat
Squamous Cell Carcinoma (SCC)		
Second most common form of skin cancer Grows more rapidly than BCC May metastasize if left untreated	Chronic sun exposure Additional risk factors same as those for BCC	Red, crusted, or nonhealing nodule or ulcer
Melanoma		
Least common skin cancer Accounts for 75% of skin cancer deaths* Elevation indicates a more	Sun exposure Fair complexion, freckling, light hair Multiple moles Male gender Familiar or personal	Brown, flat lesion with irregular borders Variegated pigmentation with poorly defined margins May begin as

Continued

TYPES OF SKIN CANCER—Cont'd

Description	Risk factors	Symptoms
Melanoma–Cont'd		
advanced stage	history of melanoma Immune suppression[†]	only 0.5-1.0 cm in diameter Changing size and shape of an existing mole Possible tenderness, bleeding, or itching

*From National Cancer Institute: SEER stat fact sheets: *Melanoma of the skin,* 2017. http://seer.cancer.gov/statfacts/html/melan.html.

[†]From American Cancer Society: *Melanoma skin cancer,* 2018. www.cancer.org/cancer/skincancer-melanoma/detailedguide/melanoma-skin-cancer-risk-factors.

From Yoost BL, Crawford LR: *Fundamentals of nursing: active learning for collaborative practice,* ed 2, St. Louis, 2020, Elsevier.

SCREENING FOR MELANOMA

A = Asymmetry	B = Border	C = Color	D = Diameter	E = Evolving
One half of lesion does not match the other half	Irregular, uneven, or notched borders	Variable in color Ranges from tan, brown, or black to white, red, or blue	Typically exceeds size of pencil eraser: >6 mm	Looks different from other moles Changes in size, shape, or color

From Yoost BL, Crawford LR: *Fundamentals of nursing: active learning for collaborative practice,* ed 2, St. Louis, 2020, Elsevier.

HAIR INSPECTION AND PALPATION
Distribution and Abnormalities

Dandruff: Overuse of products that wash away the skin's natural oils and lubricants leads to dandruff or to aggravation of underlying skin conditions, causing flakiness, dryness, and pruritus of the scalp.

Hirsutism: A condition affecting both men and women in which hair growth on the upper lip, chin, and cheeks becomes excessive, and vellus body hair becomes thicker and coarser. This condition is common in patients with hormone imbalances.

Alopecia: Permanent or temporary hair loss and extreme thinning of hair, in which the scalp is clearly visible, often is related to genetic predisposition, endocrine disorders, severe febrile illness, chemotherapy, or scalp disease.

Parasite infestation: Presence of head lice, bedbugs, or other parasitic insects may exist. Evidence of pruritus may be present from bites that are visible.

NAIL INSPECTION AND PALPATION
Capillary Refill Assessment

Measured in seconds. Blanching that occurs with pressure should reverse, with return of the nail bed to normal color in less than 2 to 3 seconds; this response is referred to as *brisk*. Capillary refill lasting longer than 2 to 3 seconds (slow or sluggish capillary refill) usually is a sign of respiratory or cardiac disease associated with hypoxia, anemia, or conditions linked to circulatory insufficiency.

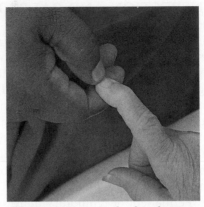

Capillary refill assessment on the hand. (From Yoost BL, Crawford LR: *Fundamentals of nursing: active learning for collaborative practice*, ed 2, St. Louis, 2020, Elsevier.)

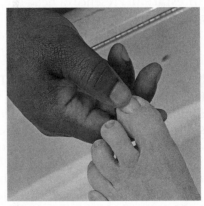

Capillary refill assessment on the large toe. (From Yoost BL, Crawford LR: *Fundamentals of nursing: active learning for collaborative practice*, ed 2, St. Louis, 2020, Elsevier.)

Nail Abnormalities

Abnormality	Cause(s)
Splinter hemorrhage: Red or purple-brown streak in nail bed	Minor trauma, trichinosis, subacute bacterial endocarditis
Paronychia: Inflammation of the skin at the base of the nail	Local infection • Acute: *Staphylococcus aureus*, herpes simplex virus • Chronic: *Candida albicans, Pseudomonas* spp.

Abnormality	Cause(s)
Clubbing: Enlargement of the fingertips, softening of the nail bed, and flattening of the nail; angle between the nail plate and the nail often greater than 180 degrees Clubbing—early Clubbing—middle Clubbing—severe almost 180° 180° >180°	Chronic hypoxia from heart and/or pulmonary disease
Beau's lines: Transverse ridging in nails due to a temporary halt in nail growth	Nail injury, systemic injury, eczema, psoriasis, paronychia

Koilonychia: Concave curves of the nail, with thinning of the nail plate; also called "spoon nail"

Iron deficiency anemia, repeated chemical trauma, syphilis

Muehrcke's lines: Double band of white lines (leukonychia)

Renal disease

From Yoost BL, Crawford LR: *Fundamentals of nursing: active learning for collaborative practice,* ed 2, St. Louis, 2020, Elsevier.

For additional information on skin, hair, and nail assessment, consult the following:

Ball JW, et al: *Seidel's guide to physical examination,* ed 9, St. Louis, 2019, Elsevier.

Jarvis C: *Physical examination and health assessment,* ed 8, St. Louis, 2020, Elsevier.

Potter PA, Perry AG, Stockert PA, Hall AM: *Fundamentals of nursing,* ed 10, St. Louis, 2021, Elsevier.

Wilson SF, Giddens JF: *Health assessment for nursing practice,* ed 6, St. Louis, 2017, Elsevier.

Yoost BL, Crawford LR: *Fundamentals of nursing: active learning for collaborative practice,* ed 2, St. Louis, 2020, Elsevier.

CHAPTER 11

Head, Eyes, Ears, Nose, and Throat Assessment (HEENT)

HEAD, EYES, EARS, NOSE, AND THROAT HEALTH ASSESSMENT QUESTIONS

Head and Neck

- Do you have a history of any head injuries (e.g., concussion), subdural hematoma, or recent lumbar punctures? Have you ever experienced dizziness or had a tumor or seizure disorder? Have you lost consciousness for any period of time or become confused and/or dazed for an unknown reason?

Do you have a history of high or low thyroid hormone levels?

- Do you have a history of headaches? If so, what are the typical onset, duration, and resolution of the headaches? Have you ever been diagnosed with migraines?
- Is there a risk of head injury in your employment? Do you wear a hard hat? Do you wear head protection when participating in sports? Do you wear a motorcycle or bicycle helmet?

Eyes

- Have you noticed any change in your vision? Have you experienced halos around lights, floaters, light sensitivity, or double vision (diplopia)?
- Do you have a history of glaucoma or cataracts? Have you ever had eye surgery?
- Do you wear contact lenses or glasses?
- Do you have any superficial or deep pain in or around the eye? Have you noticed any burning, itching, or discharge?
- When was your last eye examination?

Ears

- Do you have a history of dizziness or vertigo, earache, or hearing loss?
- Do you ever experience ringing in the ears?
- Do you wear hearing aids or use another type of hearing assistive device? Do you wear ear protection for your work?
- When was your last hearing test?

Nose

- Do you have a history of allergies, sinus infections, or trauma to the nose? Do you experience nasal discharge? If so, describe its character, including color, odor, amount, and duration.

- Do you experience sinus pain or tenderness, postnasal drip, daytime cough, headache, or face pain?
- Do you snore? If so, when is it most common for you to snore? Does it wake you or your partner? Do you feel tired after sleeping all night? Do you need frequent naps?
- Do you have a history of nosebleeds? If so, describe the frequency, amount of bleeding, and treatment.

Mouth and Throat
- Is there a personal or family history of mouth or throat cancer?
- Do you experience frequent bleeding of the gums, tooth pain, tonsillitis, cold sores, dry mouth, or cracked lips?
- Do you have any difficulty swallowing, or do you feel as though something is caught in your throat?
- When was your last dental examination?

HEAD INSPECTION AND PALPATION

Inspect head position, watching for tremors or jerking movements indicating possible neurologic disorders.

Inspect the skull for size, shape, and symmetry. Note abnormal lesions, incisions, masses, or nodules that are distinct in appearance, texture, or contour from the surrounding skin.

Inspect the size, shape, and contour of the head, and eye and ear location for symmetry.

Palpate the scalp for nodules, scars, or any abnormalities.

NORMAL EYE ANATOMY

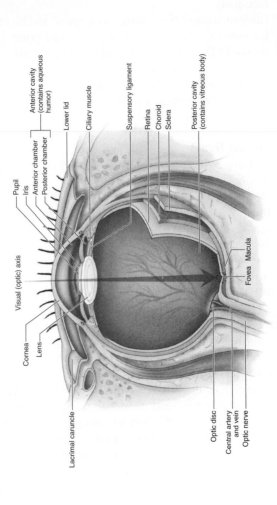

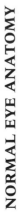

(From Patton KT, Thibodeau GA: *The human body in health and disease*, ed. 6, St. Louis, 2014, Elsevier.)

EYE INSPECTION AND PALPATION

Inspect the eyes for alignment, positioning, strabismus, protrusion, extraocular movements, and visual acuity.

Note the appearance of the sclera and conjunctiva.

Inspect the clarity of the lens and cornea.

Check pupil size, shape, and pupillary reflexes and accommodation.

Inspect the eyebrows and eyelids for position, symmetry, color, alignment, and movement.

Palpate the eyelids for nodules, and gently palpate the eye itself with the eyelids closed.

SIX FIELDS OF VISION

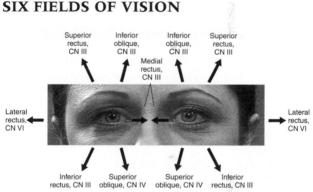

(From Ball JW, Dains JE, Flynn JA, et al.: *Seidel's guide to physical examination,* ed. 9, St. Louis, 2019, Elsevier.)

PUPILLARY SIZE CHART

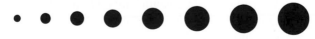

2 mm 3 mm 4 mm 5 mm 6 mm 7 mm 8 mm 9 mm

(From Yoost BL, Crawford LR: *Fundamentals of nursing: active learning for collaborative practice,* ed 2, St. Louis, 2020, Elsevier.)

ASSESSMENT OF PUPILLARY LIGHT REFLEX

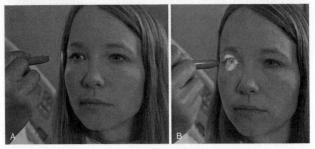

(From Yoost BL, Crawford LR: *Fundamentals of nursing: active learning for collaborative practice*, ed 2, St. Louis, 2020, Elsevier.)

   A. Assess pupillary light reflex by approaching one eye with a penlight from the side.
   B. Observe the closest pupil for immediate constriction followed by consensual constriction of the opposite pupil.

Conditions Affecting Visual Acuity

Cataracts

- Opacity or clouding of the eye lens
- Risk factors include:
  - Increasing age, female gender
  - Prolonged sun exposure
  - Cigarette smoking, alcohol, or steroid use
  - Diet low in antioxidants
- Prevention strategies include:
  - Wearing sunglasses and hats when outside
  - Quitting smoking and limiting alcohol consumption
  - Increasing intake of vitamins E and B
- Treatment is:
  - Surgery to replace the cloudy lens with a clear, artificial lens implant

Glaucoma
- Optic neuropathy, usually associated with increased intraocular pressure
- Risk factors include:
  - Increased age, African or Hispanic ancestry
  - Migraines, diabetes, low blood pressure
  - Increased intraocular pressure
  - Family history
  - Eye injury
- Prevention strategies include:
  - Having regular eye examinations by an ophthalmologist
  - Wearing protective eyewear at work, during construction projects, or while participating in sports to prevent injury
  - Limiting caffeine intake, increasing water consumption
  - Engaging in regular physical exercise
- Treatments are:
  - Medicated eyedrops to lower intraocular pressure
  - Laser or open-eye surgery

Macular Degeneration
- Deterioration of the macula, the area on the retina that is responsible for central vision, allowing for clear vision of fine details
- Risk factors include:
  - Family history, white ancestry
  - Overactive immune system causing inflammation
  - Smoking, hypertension, hypercholesterolemia
- Prevention strategies include:
  - Wearing sunglasses when outside
  - Taking dietary supplements, including vitamins E, C, B_6, and B_{12}, as well as beta carotene, zinc oxide, and copper

- Eating a healthy, well-balanced diet
- Treatments are:
  - Medication injection treatments
  - Thermal laser therapy
  - Photodynamic therapy

Myopia
- Nearsightedness, caused by a refractive error focusing objects in front of the retina
- Associated with increased risk for detached retina, glaucoma, and cataracts
- Risk factors include:
  - Familial history
- Treatment is:
  - Eyeglasses, contact lenses, or Lasik surgery

Hyperopia
- Farsightedness, caused by a refractive error focusing objects behind the retina
- Risk factors include:
  - Familial history
- Treatment is:
  - Eyeglasses, contact lenses, or Lasik surgery

Presbyopia
- Age-related loss of near vision due to increased lens rigidity
- Risk factors include:
  - Age older than 40 years
- Treatments are:
  - Reading glasses, bifocal, or progressive eyeglasses or contacts
  - Conductive keratoplasty (CK), Lasik or refractive lens exchange surgery

NORMAL EAR ANATOMY

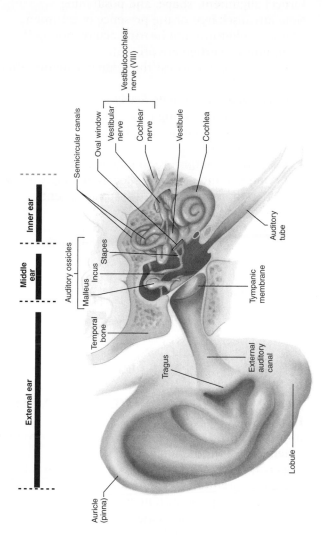

(From Patton KT, Thibodeau GA: *The human body in health and disease*, ed 6, St. Louis, 2014, Elsevier.)

EAR INSPECTION

Inspect alignment, shape, and positioning.

Note any discharge or the presence of cerumen.

Check equilibrium and hearing acuity, noting if tinnitus or vertigo are present.

Use an otoscope to assess the tympanic membrane.

Conditions Affecting Hearing Acuity

- Sensorineural hearing loss
  - Secondary to inner ear damage
- Possible causes
  - Prolonged exposure to loud sounds
  - Ototoxic medications, such as aminoglycosides, loop diuretics, and antineoplastic agents
- Conductive hearing loss
  - Secondary to interference with the transmission of sound via vibration to the inner ear
- Possible causes
  - Fluid in the middle ear
  - Cerumen accumulation
  - Atrophy of the tympanic membrane or otosclerosis in older adults
- Mixed hearing loss
  - Middle ear damage
  - Nerve damage

NOSE AND SINUS INSPECTION AND PALPATION

Inspect the nose for color, shape, symmetry, swelling, tenderness, and drainage.

Inspect the nares for swelling, color, inflammation, skin excoriation, bleeding, and polyps. If nasal discharge is present, note the character, amount, and color of the discharge and whether it is unilateral or bilateral.

Palpate the ridge and soft tissues of the nose by placing one finger on each side of the nasal arch and gently pressing the fingers from the nasal bridge to the tip of the nose. Note any displacement of bone or cartilage, tenderness, masses, or lumps.

Inspect the maxillary sinus areas (A) below the eyes for swelling and discoloration, which may be associated with a history of sinusitis, allergies, or recent viral illness.

Palpate the frontal sinuses (B) by using the thumbs to press up on the eyebrows without pushing on the eyes. Move down to both sides of the nose, and press gently with thumbs up to palpate the maxillary sinuses.

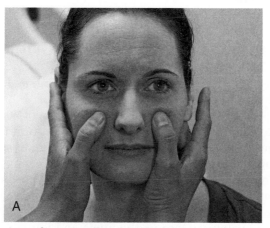

Palpating the maxillary and frontal sinus cavities. (**A**) Maxillary.

Continued

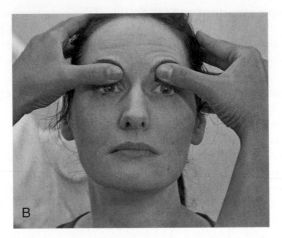

(**B**) Frontal. (From Yoost BL, Crawford LR: *Fundamentals of nursing: active learning for collaborative practice,* ed 2, St. Louis, 2020, Elsevier.)

MOUTH AND THROAT INSPECTION AND PALPATION

Inspect the lips for color, patency, scarring, and hydration.

Inspect the teeth to determine the quality of dental hygiene and the ability to chew food for nutritional intake. Inspect the teeth for color, irregular shape, and cavities (caries).

Using a tongue blade and penlight, inspect the buccal mucosa, teeth, gums, tongue, uvula, tonsils, and palate for color, texture, lesions, ulcers, bleeding, and patency. Observe the uvula and tonsils for enlargement, edema, and discoloration.

Palpate the surface of the lips and the skin around them.

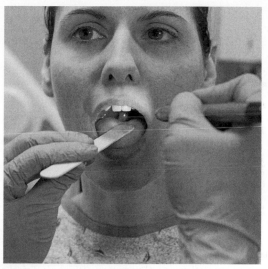

Oral cavity assessment. (From Yoost BL, Crawford LR: *Fundamentals of nursing: active learning for collaborative practice*, ed 2, St. Louis, 2020, Elsevier.)

While wearing gloves, insert the index finger into the patient's mouth and carefully palpate the gums and oral mucosa for any lesions, masses, pain, or thickening. No tenderness, bleeding, or swelling should be present. Using the 2 × 2 gauze pad, gently grasp the tongue and visualize the bottom of the mouth to check for possible lesions or abnormalities.

JAW AND LYMPH NODE INSPECTION AND PALPATION

Inspect the jaw for redness or swelling. Facing the patient, look for facial asymmetry, indicating swelling or malocclusions.

Palpate the jaw for edema or warmth.

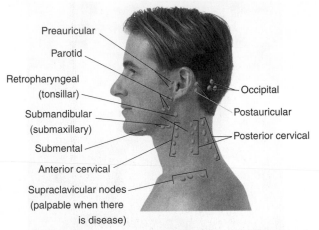

Preauricular

Parotid

Retropharyngeal
(tonsillar)

Submandibular
(submaxillary)

Submental

Anterior cervical

Supraclavicular nodes
(palpable when there
is disease)

Occipital

Postauricular

Posterior cervical

Lymphatic drainage system of head and neck. (If the group of nodes is often referred to by a second name, that name appears in parentheses.) (From Ball JW, et al.: *Seidel's guide to physical examination*, ed 9, St. Louis, 2019, Elsevier.)

Inspect the lymph nodes of the neck for symmetry and any superficial abnormalities.

Using the pads of the middle two or three fingers of both hands, gently palpate the lymph nodes on each side of the patient's neck simultaneously, comparing one side with the other. Note the size, shape, location, and consistency of any palpable nodes. Consider the warmth of the skin over the area, and note whether palpable nodes are mobile or stationary, compared with the surrounding structures.

NECK INSPECTION, PALPATION, AND AUSCULTATION

Inspect the neck for flexibility, strength, and discomfort.

Observe the jugular veins for distention and blood flow.

Note if bounding pulses are visible while inspecting the carotid arteries. Palpate only one carotid artery at a time.

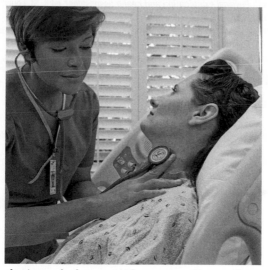

Auscultation of the carotid artery. (From Yoost BL, Crawford LR: *Fundamentals of nursing: active learning for collaborative practice,* ed 2, St. Louis, 2020, Elsevier.)

Auscultate each carotid artery for a bruit.
Inspect the thyroid gland for position and enlargement.
Palpate the trachea by feeling for the cartilage rings at the sternal notch. Tumors, thyroid gland enlargement, or conditions such as pneumothorax may cause the trachea to deviate to one side.

For additional information on HEENT assessment, consult the following:

Ball JW, et al: *Seidel's guide to physical examination,* ed 9, St. Louis, 2019, Elsevier.

Jarvis C: *Physical examination and health assessment,* ed 8, St. Louis, 2020, Elsevier.

Potter PA, Perry AG, Stockert PA, Hall AM: *Fundamentals of nursing,* ed 10, St. Louis, 2021, Elsevier.

Wilson SF, Giddens JF: *Health assessment for nursing practice,* ed 6, St. Louis, 2017, Elsevier.

Yoost BL, Crawford LR: *Fundamentals of nursing: active learning for collaborative practice,* ed 2, St. Louis, 2020, Elsevier.

CHAPTER 12

Respiratory Assessment

RESPIRATORY HEALTH ASSESSMENT QUESTIONS

- How far can you walk on level ground?
- How many stairs are you able to climb without becoming short of breath?
- Do you have a cough? If so, when did it start?
- Do you cough up mucus or blood? If so, describe the color and consistency.
- Can you lie flat when sleeping?
- Do you snore?
- Do you use oxygen or breathing machines at home? If so, how often and at what setting?
- Do you ever experience shortness of breath either at rest or with exercise?
- Do you have any pain with breathing?
- Is the pain associated with coughing, shortness of breath, trauma, nasal congestion, or sore throat?
- Does chest pain cause splinting, shallow breathing, or uneven chest expansion, or does it radiate to the back, neck, or arms?

- What relieves the chest pain associated with respiration?
- Do you have any recent history of trauma or infection?
- Do you have a history of chronic conditions that affect respiration, including allergies, emphysema, chronic obstructive pulmonary disease (COPD), tuberculosis, cystic fibrosis, or asthma?
- Do you have a history of tumors or lung cancer?
- Do you use tobacco or marijuana? If so, how often and how many years and/or packs per day?
- Have you been exposed to dust, fumes, or smoke in the environment at work or home?
- Have you traveled out of the country recently?

RESPIRATORY SYSTEM

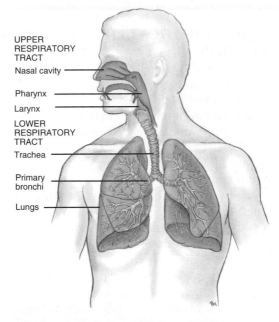

(From Applegate E: *The anatomy and physiology learning system,* ed 4, St. Louis, 2011, Elsevier.)

CHEST INSPECTION AND PALPATION

- Inspect the anterior and posterior thorax for symmetry and shape.
- Observe for the presence of a barrel chest. The anteroposterior measurement should be less than the transverse measurement.
- Inspect chest hair for color, thickness, and even distribution across the chest and upper abdomen. Nipples should be centered on either side of the sternum.
- Observe the spine, which normally is midline and straight. Ribs should slope downward, with symmetric intercostal spaces. Note any lesions, scarring, or grossly asymmetric features.

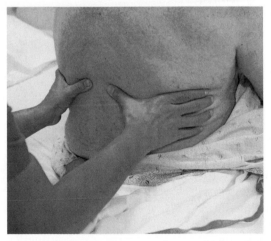

(From Yoost BL, Crawford LR: *Fundamentals of nursing: active learning for collaborative practice,* ed 2, St. Louis, 2020, Elsevier.)

- Palpate the anterior and posterior thorax to evaluate chest size, shape, and excursion. Note any superficial lumps or masses, increased skin temperature, moisture, or tenderness during palpation.
- Palpate for tactile fremitus, a palpable vibration transmitted through the chest wall that occurs with the movement of the vocal cords during speech.

BREATHING INSPECTION
- Observe chest expansion during breathing, watching for symmetry and regular, even inspiratory and expiratory effort.

Conditions Affecting Respiratory Effort
Pulmonary embolism (PE)
- Chest pain
- Shortness of breath (SOB)
- Coughing
- Diaphoresis

Cerebral palsy

Rib fracture

Severe skeletal deformities
- Kyphosis

Chronic obstructive pulmonary disease
- Emphysema
- Asthma

Disease processes
- Pneumonia
- Pleural effusion
- Pleurisy
- Bronchitis

- Pulmonary edema
- Lung cancer

Lung obstruction or collapse
- Atelectasis
- Pneumothorax
- Tumors

SIGNS AND SYMPTOMS OF HYPERVENTILATION

- Tachycardia, chest pain, shortness of breath
- Dizziness, lightheadedness, disorientation
- Paresthesia, numbness
- Tinnitus, blurred vision, tetany

SIGNS AND SYMPTOMS OF HYPOVENTILATION

- Dizziness, headache, lethargy
- Disorientation, convulsions, coma
- Decreased ability to follow directions
- Cardiac arrhythmias, electrolyte imbalance, cardiac arrest

SIGNS AND SYMPTOMS OF HYPOXIA

- Restlessness, anxiety, disorientation
- Decreased concentration, fatigue
- Decreased consciousness, dizziness
- Behavioral changes, pallor
- Increased pulse and blood pressure
- Cardiac arrhythmias, cyanosis, clubbing, dyspnea

AUSCULTATION OF THE LUNGS

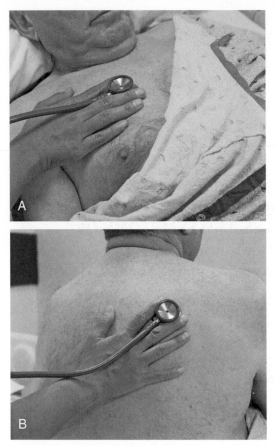

(From Yoost BL, Crawford LR: *Fundamentals of nursing: active learning for collaborative practice,* ed 2, St. Louis, 2020, Elsevier.)

- Auscultate the lungs systematically on the chest (A) and back (B) with a stethoscope placed directly on the skin. Inspiration normally is longer than expiration in adults.

Systematic Pattern for Auscultation

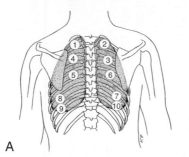

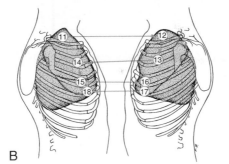

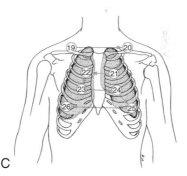

Systematic pattern for auscultation—posterior, lateral, and anterior. (From Potter PA, Perry AG, Stockert PA, Hall AM: *Fundamentals of nursing,* ed 9, St. Louis, 2017, Elsevier.)

NORMAL BREATH SOUNDS

Breath Sound	Pitch	Quality	Amplitude	Duration	Location
Tracheal	High	Harsh	Loud		Over the trachea
Bronchial	High	Hollow	Loud	Inspiration < expiration	Over the main bronchi
Bronchovesicular	Medium	Mixed	Medium	Inspiration = expiration	Posterior between the scapulae; anterior around the upper sternum in the first two intercostal spaces
Vesicular	Low	Blowing	Soft	Inspiration > expiration	Over most of the lung fields

From Yoost BL, Crawford LR: *Fundamentals of nursing: active learning for collaborative practice*, ed 2, St. Louis, 2020, Elsevier.

ADVENTITIOUS BREATH SOUNDS

Sound	Site	Cause	Character
Crackles (formerly called *rales*)	Right and left lung bases	Sudden opening of small airways and alveoli collapsed by fluid or exudate; heard in patients with cystic fibrosis, asthma, COPD, bronchitis, and pulmonary edema from left-sided heart failure	Brief crackling, popping sounds heard when a blocked airway suddenly opens; more common during inspiration; often described as fine, medium, and coarse. *Fine crackles:* Soft, high-pitched, and very brief sounds during late inspiration and not cleared by coughing *Medium crackles:* Lower-pitched, moist sounds best heard at the inspiratory midpoint

Continued

ADVENTITIOUS BREATH SOUNDS—Cont'd

Sound	Site	Cause	Character
			Coarse crackles: Loud, effervescent sounds heard best during inspiration and not relieved after coughing
Rhonchi	Over the trachea and bronchi, but can be referred to all lung fields	Increased secretions in large airways due to pneumonia; increased airway turbulence from mucus or muscle spasm	Low-pitched, snoring sounds heard either during inspiration or expiration and usually cleared with coughing; lower in pitch than wheezes, with a sonorous quality
Wheezing	All lung fields	High-velocity airflow through severely constricted or obstructed airways due to asthma, foreign objects, bronchiectasis, or emphysema	High-pitched, whistling sound heard on inspiration or expiration but most obvious and loudest during expiration; also called *sibilant wheezing*

ADVENTITIOUS BREATH SOUNDS—Cont'd

Sound	Site	Cause	Character
Stridor	Trachea and large airways	Turbulent airflow in the upper airway; may be indicative of serious airway obstruction from epiglottitis, croup, a foreign body lodged in the airway, or a laryngeal tumor	Intense, high-pitched, and continuous monophonic wheeze or crowing sound, loudest during inspiration when airways collapse owing to lower internal lumen pressure; often heard without the aid of a stethoscope
Pleural friction rub	Anterior lateral thorax	Inflamed pleural surfaces rubbing together during respiration, due to pneumonia or pleuritis	Low-pitched, grating, or creaking sound heard during inspiration or expiration and not cleared by coughing

From Yoost BL, Crawford LR: *Fundamentals of nursing: active learning for collaborative practice*, ed 2, St. Louis, 2020, Elsevier.

For additional information on respiratory assessment, consult the following:

Ball JW, et al: *Seidel's guide to physical examination,* ed 9, St. Louis, 2019, Elsevier.

Jarvis C: *Physical examination and health assessment*, ed 8, St. Louis, 2020, Elsevier.

Potter PA, Perry AG, Stockert PA, Hall AM: *Fundamentals of nursing*, ed 10, St. Louis, 2021, Elsevier.

Wilson SF, Giddens JF: *Health assessment for nursing practice,* ed 6, St. Louis, 2017, Elsevier.

Yoost BL, Crawford LR: *Fundamentals of nursing: active learning for collaborative practice,* ed 2, St. Louis, 2020, Elsevier.

CHAPTER 13

Cardiac and Peripheral Vascular Assessment

CARDIOVASCULAR HEALTH ASSESSMENT QUESTIONS

- Are you experiencing chest pain? If so, describe the pain. When was its onset, or when did the pain begin? What is its duration, or how long have you had this pain? What are the characteristics of the pain (sharp, stabbing, aching, burning, viselike)? Where is the pain? Does the pain radiate? Does anything relieve the pain? Are there any other symptoms associated with the pain?
- Do you have any palpitations or extreme fatigue?
- Do you have any difficulty breathing or difficulty lying flat when sleeping?
- Do you have any past medical history of cardiac surgery or hospitalization for cardiac events or disorders?
- Have you ever had acute rheumatic fever, swollen or painful joints, or been diagnosed with any rheumatic disorders?
- Do you have any chronic illnesses, such as hypertension, hyperlipidemia, diabetes, coronary

artery disease, congenital heart defects, or bleeding disorders?

- Do you have a family history of diabetes, heart disease, hypertension, hyperlipidemia, obesity, congenital or acquired heart defects, or sudden death at a young age? If so, include age at the time of diagnosis and death of first-degree relatives.
- Are you on an anticoagulant? Do you have a coagulation disorder?
- Does your employment include physical demands, emotional stress, or environmental hazards such as chemicals, heat, sunlight, or dust?
- Do you use tobacco? If so, at what age did you start? How many packs per day? Have you stopped using it?
- How often do you use alcohol or recreational drugs? If used, what type of alcohol or recreational drugs do you prefer?
- What is your nutritional status? Have you lost or gained weight recently?
- What do you do to relax?
- Do you exercise? How much and how often?
- Do you have aching, cramping, or pain in the legs while walking or exercising? If so, when did it start, how long have you had it, and what are its characteristics? Does anything relieve the pain?
- Have you ever lost consciousness or experienced transient syncope? If so, was the episode associated with any other symptoms?
- Does shortness of breath interfere with your activities of daily living?
- Do you have any tingling, numbness, or coldness in your hands or feet?
- Do you have edema or swelling in your hands, feet, or ankles? If so, what makes it worse? What reduces the edema?
- Have you had any recent change in hair loss or growth on your hands, feet, or ankles?
- Has anything restricted blood flow to your extremities (cast, surgery, trauma, tight clothing)?

STRUCTURE OF THE HEART

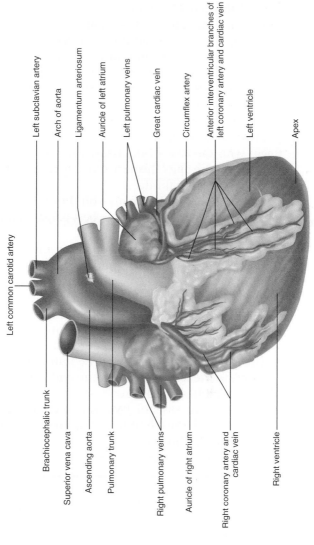

Left common carotid artery

Left subclavian artery

Arch of aorta

Ligamentum arteriosum

Auricle of left atrium

Left pulmonary veins

Great cardiac vein

Circumflex artery

Anterior interventricular branches of left coronary artery and cardiac vein

Left ventricle

Apex

Brachiocephalic trunk

Superior vena cava

Ascending aorta

Pulmonary trunk

Right pulmonary veins

Auricle of right atrium

Right coronary artery and cardiac vein

Right ventricle

(From Patton KT, Thibodeau GA: *Anatomy and physiology*, ed. 9, St. Louis, 2016, Elsevier.)

HEART INSPECTION AND PALPATION

- Assist the patient into a supine position or raise the head of the bed 45 degrees.
- Inspect and palpate in a systematic sequence according to anatomic position. Cardiac function is assessed through the anterior chest wall.
  - The right ventricle composes most of the heart's anterior surface. A portion of the left ventricle is near the fourth and fifth intercostal spaces of the anterior chest, medial to the left midclavicular line.
- Begin with the base of the heart and move in the direction of the apex. Inspect and palpate the angle of Louis and sternal ridge.
- There are anatomic landmarks on the chest wall where heart valve closures are best palpated and auscultated.
  - Find the second intercostal space on the right to locate the first of these landmarks, the aortic area.
  - The pulmonic region can be found at the second or third intercostal space on the left.
  - The tricuspid area is found at the fourth or fifth intercostal space, along the sternum.
  - The mitral area is located at the fifth intercostal space, to the left of the sternum, and laterally to the left midclavicular line.
  - The apical impulse, or PMI, is located in the mitral area at the left fifth intercostal space at the midclavicular line. The PMI is felt as a brief pulsation in the area 1 to 2 cm (1/2 to 3/4 inch) around the region of the apex. It is not uncommon to visualize the apical impulse when the patient sits up, because the heart moves closer to the anterior chest wall.

- The final anatomic landmark is the epigastric area just below the tip of the sternum. The abdominal aorta is in the upper midline abdomen, 2 to 3 inches above the umbilicus and below the xiphoid process.
  - Palpate the abdominal aorta by applying gentle, downward pressure with the flattened fingers of both hands to indent the epigastrium toward the spine.
  - In extremely obese people or in those with very developed abdominal musculature, aortic pulsation may not be detected.
  - Bounding aortic pulsations may indicate an abdominal aortic aneurysm.

AUSCULTATION OF THE HEART

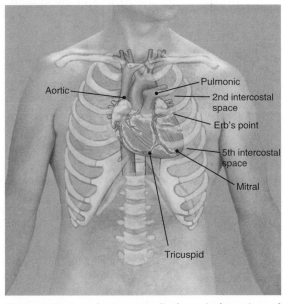

(In Linton AD: *Introduction to medical-surgical nursing*, ed. 5, St. Louis, 2012, Saunders. From Monahan FD, Drake DT, Neighbors M, eds: *Medical-surgical nursing: Foundations for clinical practice*, ed. 2, Philadelphia, 1998, Saunders.)

- In a quiet environment, auscultate for the complete cycle of heart sounds ("lub-dub") using the diaphragm first and then the bell of the stethoscope at each of the anatomical sites associated with cardiac valves and blood flow.
  - Isolate each sound, listening for as many beats as necessary to evaluate the sounds. Glide the stethoscope systematically through each of the anatomical areas in a sequence moving from the base to the apex of the heart. Breast tissue may need to be gently moved to allow heart sounds to be heard more clearly.
  - Use firm pressure with the diaphragm and light pressure with the bell for better auscultation of heart murmurs. Usually, auscultation in all areas is performed with the patient in the supine, sitting, and left lateral recumbent positions if the patient's condition permits.
- On auscultation, two distinct heart sounds are heard, S1 ("lub") and S2 ("dub"). An entire S1 plus S2 ("lub-dub") cycle constitutes one heartbeat.
  - S1 is the sound of the mitral and tricuspid valves closing and marks the beginning of systole. The S1 sound is dull and low-pitched and is heard best at the apex of the heart. It should coordinate with carotid artery pulsation.
  - S2 is the sound of the aortic and pulmonic valves closing and marks the end of systole and the beginning of diastole. It is best heard in the aortic region.
- In some cases, rapid ventricular filling creates a third heart sound, S3 ("lub-dub-dub"), which is heard more often in children and adolescent patients. Presence of an S3 sound usually is a benign condition that the affected person outgrows as the cardiac vasculature becomes thicker and stronger. An S3 murmur is considered abnormal in adults older than 25 to 30 years of age.

- When atria contract to enhance ventricular filling, a fourth heart sound, S4, is created. It is heard just before S1 ("lub-lub-dub"). An S4 heart sound is not a normal finding in adults, but it can be heard in healthy older adults, children, and athletes. Because it may indicate an abnormal condition, the presence of an S4 heart sound should be documented and reported to the patient's primary care provider.
- A new onset of S4, a pulse deficit, or extra heart sounds should be reported to the patient's primary care provider for further investigation.

PERIPHERAL VASCULAR INSPECTION AND PALPATION

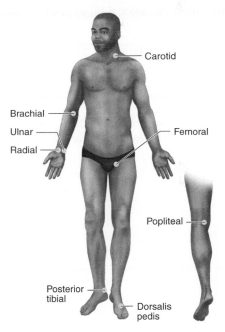

(From Yoost BL, Crawford LR: *Fundamentals of nursing: active learning for collaborative practice,* ed 2, St. Louis, 2020, Elsevier.)

- Assess arterial pulses in all superficial locations using the fingertips of the first three fingers.
  - Note intensity, rate, rhythm, existence of blood vessel tenderness, tortuosity, or nodularity.
  - Inspection of the skin and nails may also indicate arterial or venous impairment.
- Palpation of the brachial, radial, ulnar, femoral, popliteal, dorsalis pedis, and posterior tibial arteries is done using the fingertips.
- Compare peripheral pulses side to side for strength and symmetry.
- Intensity or volume of peripheral pulses is graded on a scale of 0 to 3:

0	Absent pulse (unable to palpate)
1	Diminished (weaker than expected; difficult to palpate)
2	Normal (able to palpate with normal pressure)
3	Bounding (may be able to see pulsation; doesn't disappear with palpation)

- A handheld Doppler ultrasound is used to further assess weak or seemingly absent peripheral pulses.

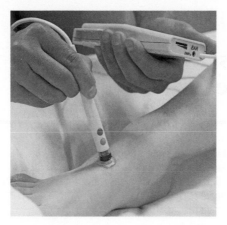

(From Yoost BL, Crawford LR: *Fundamentals of nursing: active learning for collaborative practice,* ed 2, St. Louis, 2020, Elsevier.)

For additional information on cardiovascular assessment, consult the following:

Ball JW, et al: *Seidel's guide to physical examination,* ed 9, St. Louis, 2019, Elsevier.

Jarvis C: *Physical examination and health assessment,* ed 8, St. Louis, 2020, Elsevier.

Potter PA, Perry AG, Stockert PA, Hall AM: *Fundamentals of nursing,* ed 10, St. Louis, 2021, Elsevier.

Wilson SF, Giddens JF: *Health assessment for nursing practice,* ed 6, St. Louis, 2017, Elsevier.

Yoost BL, Crawford LR: *Fundamentals of nursing: active learning for collaborative practice,* ed 2, St. Louis, 2020, Elsevier.

CHAPTER 14

Musculoskeletal Assessment

MUSCULOSKELETAL HEALTH ASSESSMENT QUESTIONS

- Do you have any pain or stiffness in your joints, muscles, or back? If so, when did it begin? Where is the pain or stiffness? What is its quality? Is the pain burning, aching, shooting, constant, or intermittent? Does anything aggravate or relieve the pain?
- Are you able to perform activities of daily living, such as dressing or preparing meals, without musculoskeletal discomfort?
- Can you climb stairs and walk without limping?
- Do you have numbness or tingling in your extremities?
- Are you able to engage in strenuous activity or exercise?
- Have you experienced any recent trauma to any of your bones, joints, soft tissue, or nerves?
- Do you have any chronic illnesses that may affect the musculoskeletal system, including cancer, osteoporosis, arthritis, and renal or neurological disorders?

- Do you have any known skeletal deformities or a congenital history that may affect the musculoskeletal system?
- Do you have any family history of arthritis (rheumatoid, osteoarthritis, ankylosing spondylitis), back problems (scoliosis, spina bifida), or genetic disorders (osteogenesis imperfecta, rickets, dwarfing syndrome)?
- Does your diet include adequate calcium and vitamin D?

MUSCULOSKELETAL INSPECTION AND PALPATION

- Inspect gait, bone alignment, function of muscles and joints.
- Observe for parallel alignment of the hips.
- Observe body symmetry.
- Check spinal alignment.

Possible Spinal Abnormalities

- Lordosis
- Kyphosis
- Scoliosis
- Osteoporosis

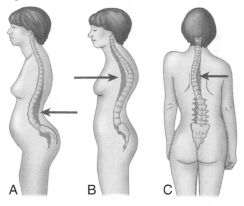

Abnormal curvatures of the spine: **(A)** lordosis; **(B)** kyphosis; and **(C)** scoliosis. (From Patton KT, Thibodeau GA: *The human body in health and disease,* ed 6, St. Louis, 2014, Elsevier.)

- Assess mobility of joints through either active or passive range of motion.

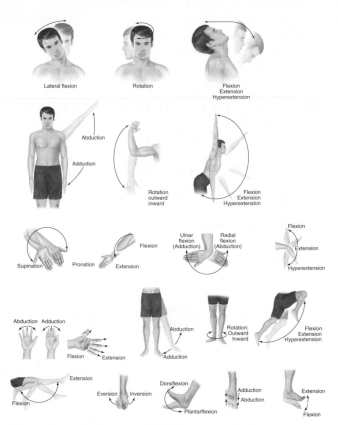

(From Yoost BL, Crawford LR: *Fundamentals of nursing: active learning for collaborative practice,* ed 2, St. Louis, 2020, Elsevier.)

DEEP AND CUTANEOUS TENDON REFLEX ASSESSMENT

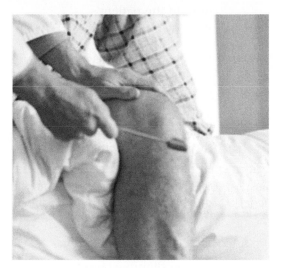

Assessment of the patellar reflex. (© Thinkstock.com.)

Reflex	Technique	Normal Response
Biceps	Place your thumb on the base of the biceps tendon in the antecubital fossa of the patient's partially flexed arm. Tap your thumb with a reflex hammer.	Biceps contraction and flexion
Triceps	Hold the upper arm of the patient at a 45-degree angle away from the patient's	Extension of the forearm

Continued

Reflex	Technique	Normal Response
	body, while it is limp, or hold the patient's wrist across the patient's chest for flexion. Tap the triceps tendon just above the elbow.	
Quadriceps or patellar knee jerk	Allow the patient's leg to dangle freely. Tap the quadriceps tendon just below the patella.	Extension of the leg
Achilles ankle jerk	Hold the patient's dorsiflexed foot with the leg flexed and the hip externally rotated. Tap the Achilles tendon slightly above and behind the inner heel area.	Plantar flexion of the foot
Plantar	With the patient lying in supine position, stroke the bottom of the patient's foot gently from the heel to the toes, in the shape of an upside-down J, ending below the big toe.	Adults and children: Plantar flexion of the toes and forefoot Infants: Dorsiflexion of the big toe and fanning out of the toes (positive Babinski sign)

From Yoost BL, Crawford LR: *Fundamentals of nursing: active learning for collaborative practice,* ed 2, St. Louis, 2020, Elsevier.

REFLEX RESPONSES

4+	Very brisk, hyperactive with clonus
3+	Brisker than average, slightly hyperactive
2+	Average, normal
1+	Sluggish or diminished
0	No response

From Yoost BL, Crawford LR: *Fundamentals of nursing: active learning for collaborative practice,* ed 2, St. Louis, 2020, Elsevier.

TYPES OF FRACTURES
Closed simple: Fracture does not break skin.
Comminuted: Bone is splintered into fragments.
Compression: Caused by compressive force; common in lumbar vertebrae.
Depressed: Broken skull bone driven inward.
Displaced: Fracture produces fragments that become misaligned.
Greenstick: Fracture in which one side of bone is broken and other side is bent.
Impacted telescoped: Bone is broken and wedged into another break.
Incomplete: Continuity of the bone has not been completely destroyed.
Longitudinal: Break runs parallel with the bone.
Oblique: Fracture line runs at a 45-degree angle across the longitudinal axis.
Open compound: Fracture breaks through skin (can be categorized into grades 1–4 depending on severity).
Pathologic: A disease process weakens bone structure so that a slight degree of trauma can cause fracture (most common in osteoporosis and cancers of the bone).

Segmental: Fracture in two places (also called double fracture).

Silver-fork: Fracture of lower end of radius.

Spiral: Break coils around the bone; can be caused by a twisting force.

Transverse: Fracture breaks across the bone at a 90-degree angle along the longitudinal axis.

For additional information on musculoskeletal assessment, consult the following:

Ball JW, et al: *Seidel's guide to physical examination,* ed 9, St. Louis, 2019, Elsevier.

Jarvis C: *Physical examination and health assessment,* ed 8, St. Louis, 2020, Elsevier.

Potter PA, Perry AG, Stockert PA, Hall AM: *Fundamentals of nursing,* ed 10, St. Louis, 2021, Elsevier.

Wilson SF, Giddens JF: *Health assessment for nursing practice,* ed 6, St. Louis, 2017, Elsevier.

Yoost BL, Crawford LR: *Fundamentals of nursing: active learning for collaborative practice,* 2e, St. Louis, 2020, Elsevier.

CHAPTER 15

Neurological Assessment

NEUROLOGICAL HEALTH ASSESSMENT QUESTIONS

- Do you have any weakness, tremors, numbness, or tingling in your arms or legs?
- Are you experiencing a loss of balance or difficulty walking?
- How would you describe your mood? Do you ever feel nervous, anxious, depressed, or confused?
- Have you noticed any problems with remembering?
- Have you ever had trauma to the head, spinal cord, or back?
- Do you have a history of meningitis or encephalitis?

- Have you ever had circulatory problems, an aneurysm, or a stroke?
- Do you have a history of seizures or convulsions? If so, when did they first occur? Describe what happens when the seizures occur. Are you on anticonvulsant medications?
- Are you having any pain? If so, where? Describe the pain.
- Do you have headaches? If so, what do they feel like?
- Do you have any dizziness, light-headedness, or fainting spells?
- Do you have any weakness or paresthesia?
- Are you having any problems with coordination or balance?
- Is there a family history of any neurological disorders?
- Have you ever been diagnosed with a learning disability?
- List any medical or metabolic disturbances, such as thyroid disease, diabetes mellitus, and hypertension.
- Do you use alcohol, recreational drugs, or prescription drugs that have mood-altering effects?
- Are you exposed to environmental or occupational hazards, such as exposure to lead, insecticides, organic cleaning solvents, arsenic, or other chemicals?

FUNCTIONS OF EACH AREA OF THE BRAIN

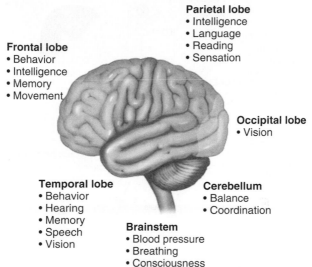

Parietal lobe
- Intelligence
- Language
- Reading
- Sensation

Frontal lobe
- Behavior
- Intelligence
- Memory
- Movement

Occipital lobe
- Vision

Temporal lobe
- Behavior
- Hearing
- Memory
- Speech
- Vision

Cerebellum
- Balance
- Coordination

Brainstem
- Blood pressure
- Breathing
- Consciousness
- Heartbeat
- Swallowing

(From Patton KT, Thibodeau GA: *The human body in health and disease,* ed 6, St. Louis, 2014, Elsevier.)

CRANIAL NERVES

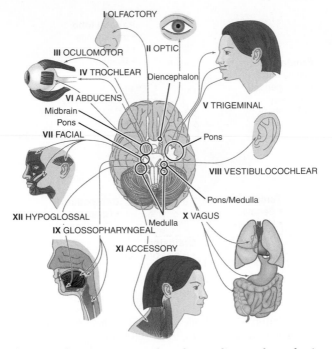

The cranial nerves are numbered according to the order in which they leave the brain. (Redrawn from McCance, KL, Huether, SE: *Pathophysiology: The biologic basis for disease in adults and children*, ed. 8, St. Louis, 2019, Elsevier.)

CRANIAL NERVE FUNCTION AND ASSESSMENT

Origin	Function	Assessment	Symptoms of Damage
Cranial Nerve I: Olfactory (Sensory)			
Upper nasal passages	Transmits the sense of smell	After assessing patency of both nares, have the patient close the eyes, obstruct one nares, and inhale to identify a common scent.	Bilateral decreased sense of smell occurs with age, tobacco smoking, allergic or chronic rhinitis, overexposure to chemical substances, and cocaine use. Unilateral loss of sense of smell can indicate a frontal lobe lesion.

Continued

CRANIAL NERVE FUNCTION AND ASSESSMENT—Cont'd

Origin	Function	Assessment	Symptoms of Damage
Cranial Nerve II: Optic (Sensory)			
Eyes	Transmits visual information to the brain; located in the optic canal	Check visual acuity (have the patient read newspaper print or use a Snellen chart), and test visual fields for each eye.	Unilateral blindness can indicate a lesion or pressure in the globe or on the optic nerve. Loss of the same half of visual field in both eyes can indicate a lesion of the opposite-side optic tract, as in a cerebrovascular accident (CVA).

Cranial Nerve III: Oculomotor (Motor)

Midbrain	Innervates four of the six muscles that collectively execute most eye movements; responsible for papillary constriction and dilation	Assess pupil size and light reflex; note direction of gaze.	A unilaterally dilated pupil with unilateral absent light reflex and/or an eye that will not gaze upward can indicate an internal carotid aneurysm or increased intracranial pressure.

Cranial Nerve IV: Trochlear (Motor)

Midbrain	Innervates muscles responsible for downward and inward gaze of the eyes	Ask the patient to gaze downward, temporally and nasally. (Note: Cranial nerves III, IV, and VI are examined together because they control eyelid elevation, eye movement, and pupillary constriction.)	If the eyes will not move through the inward and downward gazes, the patient may have a fracture of the eye orbit or a brainstem tumor.

Continued

CRANIAL NERVE FUNCTION AND ASSESSMENT—Cont'd

Origin	Function	Assessment	Symptoms of Damage
Cranial Nerve V: Trigeminal (Sensory and Motor)			
Pons	Is responsible for the corneal reflex; receives sensation from the face and innervates the muscles of mastication	Motor: Palpate jaws and temples while patient clenches teeth. Sensory: With the patient's eyes closed, gently touch a cotton ball to all areas of the face.	Unilateral deficit is seen with trauma and tumors.
Cranial Nerve VI: Abducens (Motor)			
Pons	Innervates muscles responsible for outward gaze of the eyes	Assess directions of gaze.	Inability to gaze outward may indicate a fracture of an orbit or a brainstem tumor.

Cranial Nerve VII: Facial (Sensory and Motor)

Pons	Provides motor innervation to the muscles of facial expression; receives the sense of taste from the anterior two-thirds of the tongue; provides innervation to the salivary glands (except parotid) and the lacrimal gland	Motor: Check symmetry of the face by having the patient frown, close eyes, lift eyebrows, and puff cheeks. Sensory: Assess the patient's ability to recognize taste (sugar, salt, lemon juice).	An asymmetric deficit can be found in traumatic injury, Bell's palsy, CVA, tumor, and inflammation.

Cranial Nerve VIII: Vestibulocochlear or Auditory-Vestibular (Sensory)

Medulla oblongata	Vestibular branch: Carries impulses for equilibrium Cochlear branch: Carries impulses for hearing	Assess the patient's ability to hear a spoken and whispered word.	Impairment may result from inflammation or occlusion of the ear canal, infection, drug toxicity, or a possible tumor, or may cause vertigo.

Continued

CRANIAL NERVE FUNCTION AND ASSESSMENT—Cont'd

Origin	Function	Assessment	Symptoms of Damage
Cranial Nerve IX: Glossopharyngeal (Sensory and Motor)			
Medulla oblongata	Receives taste from the posterior third of the tongue; provides innervation to the parotid gland; and provides motor innervation for swallowing	Sensory: Assess the patient's ability to taste sour or sweet on last two-thirds of tongue. Motor: Check for presence of the gag reflex by inserting a tongue blade two-thirds into the pharynx.	Deficits in taste or gag reflex can indicate a brainstem tumor or neck injury.
Cranial Nerve X: Vagus (Sensory and Motor)			
Medulla oblongata	Supplies innervation to the larynx and soft palate responsible for speech and swallowing; provides parasympathetic fibers to nearly all thoracic and abdominal smooth muscles	Depress the tongue with a tongue blade and have the patient say "ah" or yawn. The uvula and soft palate should rise and be symmetric. Assess speech for hoarseness.	Dysphagia can indicate swallowing problems and the potential for aspiration.

Cranial Nerve XI: Spinal Accessory (Motor)

Medulla oblongata (cranial root) and spinal cord (spinal root)	Cranial root: Works with vagus nerve to control the muscles of the soft palate, pharynx, and larynx Spinal root: Innervates muscles of the neck and back	Have the patient rotate the head and shrug the shoulders against passive resistance.	If the patient is unable to perform a shoulder shrug or head rotation, this may indicate a neck injury.

Cranial Nerve XII: Hypoglossal (Motor)

Medulla oblongata	Provides motor innervation to muscles of the tongue not innervated by the vagus nerve and to other glossal muscles; is important for swallowing and speech articulation	Assess tongue control (e.g., have the patient stick out the tongue and move it from side to side).	Inability to stick out the tongue may be associated with swallowing or articulation difficulties.

From Yoost BL, Crawford LR: *Fundamentals of nursing: active learning for collaborative practice*, ed 2, St. Louis, 2020, Elsevier.

SENSORY NERVE ASSESSMENT
Sensory Focused Health Assessment Questions
- Can you feel the difference between hot and cold water?
- Have you ever had a sore on your leg or foot that wouldn't heal?
- Do you have any pain, numbness, or tingling in your hands, legs, or feet?
- Are you able to smell different foods?
- Can you taste salty foods? Sweet? Sour?
- Have you noticed changes in your hearing?
- Have you ever had a hearing examination?
- Do you wear hearing aids?
- Do you ever lose your balance or feel like the room is spinning?
- When was your last eye examination?
- Do you wear glasses or contacts?
- Can you see to read the newspaper?
- Can you see objects to your left and to your right?
- Is your vision blurry?

Sensory Nerve Pathways
Dermatomes are areas of the skin that correspond to the sensory pathways that detect and conduct sensations of pain, temperature, vibration, position, and touch. Sensory receptors transmit messages to the spinal cord, from which they then travel to the brain to be interpreted.
- Check the patient's ability to identify dull and sharp sensory stimuli equally on both sides of the body.
- Ask the patient to describe the quality of each stimulus and note the presence or absence of bilateral symmetry when the stimuli are applied to the patient's extremities and trunk.
- Compare distal with proximal sensations.

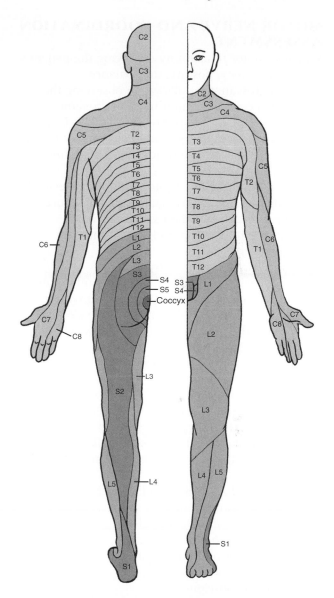

Dermatomes. (From Linton AD: *Introduction to medical-surgical nursing,* ed 5, St. Louis, 2012, Saunders.)

MOTOR NERVE AND COORDINATION ASSESSMENT

- Assess motor function by observing the patient's muscle activity, posture, and balance.
- Assess gross motor skills while observing the patient's ease and smoothness of movement.
- Assess upper extremity fine motor skills by having the patient turn pages of a book, transfer objects from one hand to the other, or write a short sentence.
- Lower extremity fine motor skills are assessed by having the patient tap each foot in quick, successive movements against the examiner's hand.
  - Test each foot separately to evaluate for symmetry.
- Balance can be assessed by:
  - Performing a Romberg test for equilibrium
    - Patients should be able to stand with their eyes closed, with arms at their sides and feet together for at least 20 seconds without losing their balance.
  - Asking the patient to stand on one foot with eyes closed
    - Patients should be able to stand on one foot with their eyes closed for at least 5 seconds.
  - Having patients walk in a straight line heel to toe
    - Patients should be able to walk in a straight line without losing their balance.

MENTAL STATUS ASSESSMENT

- Vital to determine a patient's ability to understand instructions and make decisions.
- Assess brain function related to:
  - Orientation and mental status
    - Questions
  - Level of consciousness
    - Glasgow coma scale

Orientation and Mental Status Questions
- Person: "What is your full name?"
- Place: "Where are you?"
- Time: "What (day, month, season, or year) is it?"
- Situation: "What happened that caused you to come to the hospital?"

Glasgow Coma Scale

Response	Level of Arousal	Scoring (Points)
Eye opening	Spontaneous	4
	To verbal command	3
	To pain	2
	None	1
Verbal	Oriented	5
	Confused but able to answer questions	4
	Inappropriate responses, words discernible	3
	Incomprehensible speech	2
	None	1
Motor	Obeys commands	6
	Purposeful movement to painful stimulus	5
	Withdraws from pain	4
	Abnormal (spastic) flexion, decorticate posture	3
	Extensor (rigid) response, decerebrate posture	2
	None	1
	Possible total score range	**3-15**

COGNITIVE FUNCTION ASSESSMENT
Cognition Focused Health Assessment Questions
- Do you have trouble sleeping, or do you sleep too much?
- Have you noticed difficulty adding numbers or doing your banking?
- Are you able to have conversations with others, either in person or on the phone?
- Are you able to drive to the store or do errands?
- Do you ever feel sad?
- Do you read the newspaper?
- Do you live with anyone? If so, with whom?
- What medication do you take every day?

Cognitive Physical Assessment Concerns
When sudden changes in behavior or cognitive changes are exhibited:
- Check electrolyte levels, especially sodium and calcium for both high and low levels.
- Review the patient's complete blood count (CBC) for signs of infection.
- Monitor blood glucose levels for hyperglycemia or hypoglycemia.
- Examine urinalysis findings for a possible urinary tract infection (UTI).
- Determine whether the patient has been diagnosed with an illness or experienced a trauma that involves the central nervous system.
- Evaluate the patient's ability to communicate.
- Check patient's hearing, vision, touch, smell, and taste.
- Assess the patient's ability to perform activities of daily living (ADLs).

EMOTIONAL ASSESSMENT

- Describe the patient's physical appearance, facial expression, behavior, and mood.
- What are the patient's posture and gait?
- Can the patient sit still? Is the patient experiencing tremors or muscle tension?
- Does the patient appear to be depressed or withdrawn?
- Is the patient agitated, aggressive, or angry?
- What are the patient's vital signs? Are the patient's heart rate and blood pressure elevated? Are the patient's respirations shallow? Does the patient report any pain?
- Is the patient experiencing any shortness of breath, dry mouth, or gastrointestinal upset?

Stress and Coping Health Assessment Topics and Questions

Present Stressors

- What personal stress are you currently experiencing?
- Have you experienced any changes in your life recently?
- Have you experienced changes in your stress level due to these changes?

Coping Skills

- How have you dealt with stressful situations in the past?
- Were these techniques of handling stress effective?
- Whom can you ask for assistance during stressful times?

Symptoms of Stressors

- Are you experiencing feelings of anxiety or nervousness?

- Are you experiencing feelings of depression, irritability, or anger?
- Are you experiencing your heart racing and pounding?
- Have you experienced episodes of hyperventilating?
- Does stress cause you to experience muscle tension in your neck, back, and head?
- Do you experience migraine headaches when you are under stress?
- Have you experienced diarrhea or constipation during stressful times?
- Are you having trouble sleeping?
- Have you had any changes in weight?

Adults
- Have you recently experienced any social, physical, emotional, or financial losses?
- Do you feel safe in your home?
- Do you suffer from physical illnesses?
- Have there been any major changes in your life recently?

Children
- What has been bothering you lately?
- Do you have any specific concerns?
- Do you feel safe at home and school?

Support Network
- Whom do you turn to when you need help?
- Whom do you talk to about your feelings and problems?

Additional Considerations

- Does your cultural or spiritual background provide you with certain beliefs that are helpful in times of stress?
- Do you see someone other than a doctor or nurse for health care, such as a psychologist, social worker, faith healer, folk healer, or medicine man?

Fight-or-Flight Response

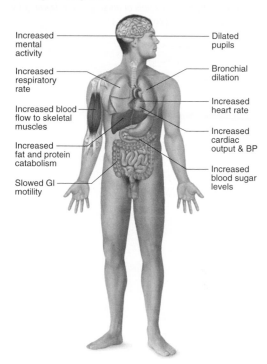

Increased mental activity

Increased respiratory rate

Increased blood flow to skeletal muscles

Increased fat and protein catabolism

Slowed GI motility

Dilated pupils

Bronchial dilation

Increased heart rate

Increased cardiac output & BP

Increased blood sugar levels

For additional information on neurological assessment,
consult the following:

Ball JW, et al: *Seidel's guide to physical examination,* ed 9, St. Louis, 2019, Elsevier.

Jarvis C: *Physical examination and health assessment,* ed 8, St. Louis, 2020, Elsevier.

Potter PA, Perry AG, Stockert PA, Hall AM: *Fundamentals of nursing,* ed 10, St. Louis, 2021, Elsevier.

Wilson SF, Giddens JF: *Health assessment for nursing practice,* ed 6, St. Louis, 2017, Elsevier.

Yoost BL, Crawford LR: *Fundamentals of nursing: active learning for collaborative practice,* 2e, St. Louis, 2021, Elsevier.

CHAPTER 16

Abdominal Assessment

ABDOMINAL HEALTH ASSESSMENT QUESTIONS
Gastrointestinal Tract

- Do you have any pain or difficulty with swallowing?
- Have you had trouble eating, weight change, or lack of appetite?
- Do you have nausea, vomiting, regurgitation of food, heartburn, indigestion, or bloating? If so, what do you do to relieve the symptoms?
- Are you experiencing abdominal pain? If so, what are the characteristics of the pain? Are there any associated symptoms? Does anything relieve the pain?
- What is your typical 24-hour food intake?
- Have you experienced any changes in bowel habits: diarrhea, constipation, incontinence, or frequent passing of gas?

- Have you noticed any blood in your stool?
- Do you have problems with hemorrhoids?
- Have you ever had abdominal surgery?
- Do you or any family members have a history of abdominal illnesses such as gallbladder disease, cancer, or irritable bowel syndrome?

Urinary Tract

- Are you experiencing any difficulty with urination: frequency or difficulty starting or stopping your stream of urine?
- Do you have a history of urinary tract or kidney infections or kidney stones?
- Do you have any pain or burning when you urinate?
- Have you noticed a change in your frequency of urination: less often or more often than previously?
- Do you feel that you empty your bladder when you urinate?
- Do you have to get up at night to urinate? If so, how many times?

GASTROINTESTINAL SYSTEM

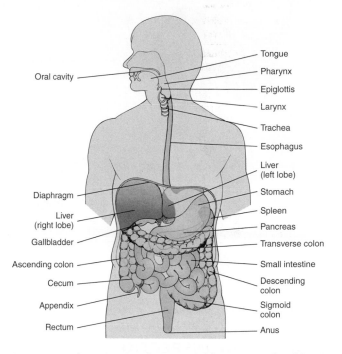

Tongue
Pharynx
Epiglottis
Larynx
Trachea
Esophagus
Liver
(left lobe)
Oral cavity
Stomach
Diaphragm
Spleen
Liver
(right lobe)
Pancreas
Gallbladder
Transverse colon
Ascending colon
Small intestine
Cecum
Descending
colon
Appendix
Sigmoid
colon
Rectum
Anus

(From Monahan FD, Sands JK, Neighbors M, et al.: *Phipps'
medical-surgical nursing: Health and illness perspectives,* ed 8,
St. Louis, 2007, Elsevier.)

URINARY SYSTEM

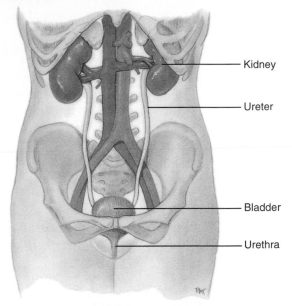

Kidney

Ureter

Bladder

Urethra

(From Applegate E: *The anatomy and physiology learning system*, ed 4, St. Louis, 2011, Elsevier.)

ABDOMINAL INSPECTION, AUSCULTATION, AND PALPATION

- Inspect the abdomen first, followed immediately by auscultation.
  - Auscultation must be completed before palpation and percussion, because pressure on the abdomen disturbs the gastrointestinal tract, altering the occurrence and character of bowel sounds.
- Note color, tone, scars, bruises, lesions, venous patterns, striae, drains, tubes, and stomas.
- Assess for distention or bulges possibly caused by flatus, ascites, tumors, hernias, or bladder distention.
- Watch for abnormal pulsations or movement, which may indicate the presence of an abdominal aortic aneurysm.

- Auscultate for bowel sounds in all four quadrants of the abdomen, which typically occur irregularly every 2 to 5 seconds. It may take up to 30 seconds to auscultate bowel sounds in all areas.
- Verify total absence of bowel sounds by listening for 5 minutes in each quadrant.
- Palpate each quadrant systematically to note tenderness, spasms or rigidity, guarding, or rebound tenderness.

Abdominal Quadrants

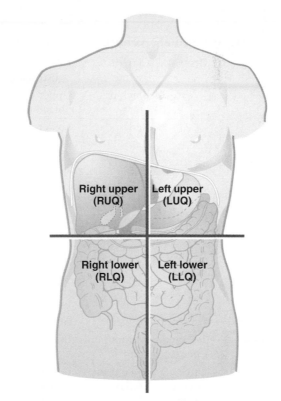

(From Black JM, Hawks JH: *Medical-surgical nursing: clinical management for positive outcomes*, ed 8, St. Louis, 2009, Elsevier.)

Conditions Affecting Bowel Elimination
- Constipation
- Impaction
- Diarrhea
- Incontinence
- Abdominal distention
- Intussusception
- Obstruction
- Paralytic ileus

FECAL CHARACTERISTICS

Characteristic	Normal	Abnormal	Assess for
Color	Brown	Clay or white	Bile obstruction
		Black or tarry	Upper GI bleeding, iron
		Red	Lower GI bleeding, beets
		Pale	Malabsorption of fat
		Green	Infection
Consistency	Moist	Hard	Constipation, dehydration
	Formed	Loose	Diet, diarrhea, medications
		Watery	Infection
		Liquid	Impaction
Odor	Aromatic	Pungent	Infection, blood
Frequency	1-2 times per day	5 times per day	Infection, diet
	Once every 3 days	Once every 6 days	Constipation, activity, medications
Shape	Cylindric	Narrow, "ribbonlike"	Obstruction

TYPES OF COMMON BOWEL OSTOMIES
Ileostomy

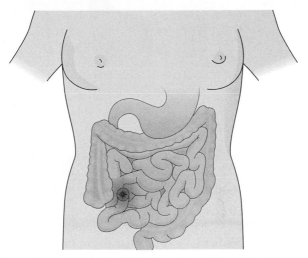

(From Perry AG, et al: *Clinical nursing skills and techniques*, ed 9, St. Louis, 2018, Elsevier.)

Drainage characteristics: A continuous discharge that is soft and wet. The output is somewhat odorous and contains intestinal enzymes that are irritating to peristomal skin.

Skin barrier option: Highly desirable for peristomal skin protection.

Pouch option: Pouch necessary at all times.

Type of pouch: Drainable or closed-end for specific needs.

Need for irrigation: None.

Transverse Colostomy

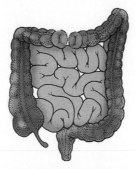

(From Ignatavicius DD, Workman ML, Rebar CR, et al.: *Medical surgical nursing: concepts for interprofessional collaborative care,* ed 9, St. Louis, 2018, Elsevier.)

Drainage characteristics: Usually semiliquid or very soft. Occasionally transverse colostomy discharge is firm. Output is usually malodorous and can irritate peristomal skin. Double-barreled colostomies have two openings. Loop colostomies have one opening but two tracks—the active (proximal), which discharges fecal matter, and the inactive (distal), which discharges mucus.

Skin barrier option: Highly desirable for peristomal skin protection.

Pouch option: Pouch necessary at all times.

Type of pouch: Drainable or closed end for specific needs.

Need for irrigation: None.

Descending Colostomy and Sigmoid Colostomy

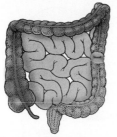
The **descending colostomy**
is done for left-sided tumors.

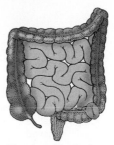
The **sigmoid colostomy**
is done for rectal tumors.

(From Ignatavicius DD, Workman ML, Rebar CR, et al.:
*Medical surgical nursing: concepts for interprofessional
collaborative care*, ed 9, St. Louis, 2018, Elsevier.)

Drainage characteristics: Semisolid from
descending colostomy. Firm from sigmoid
colostomy. On discharge, there is an odor.
Discharge is irritating if left in contact with skin
around stoma. Frequency of output is
unpredictable and varies with each person.

Skin barrier option: May be used for peristomal skin
protection if pouch is worn.

Pouch option: Pouch should be worn if person does
not irrigate.

Type of pouch: Drainable, closed-end, or stoma cap.

Need for irrigation: Yes, as instructed by
enterostomal (ET) nurse or physician.

Continent Ileostomy

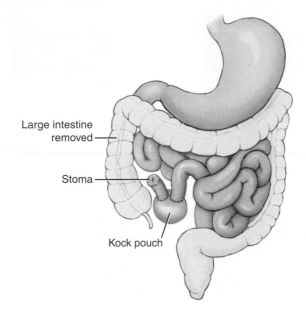

Large intestine removed

Stoma

Kock pouch

(From Potter PA, Perry AG, Stockert PA, Hall AM: *Clinical companion for fundamentals of nursing: just the facts,* ed 9, St. Louis, 2017, Elsevier.)

Drainage characteristics: Fluid bowel secretions are collected in a reservoir surgically constructed out of the lower part of the small intestine. Gas and feces are emptied via a surgically created leak-free nipple valve through which a catheter is inserted into the reservoir. For maximum efficiency and comfort, the reservoir is usually emptied four or five times daily. Daily schedule for catheterization should be recommended by the ET nurse or physician.

Skin barrier option: None; an absorbent pad provides peristomal skin protection.

Pouch option: None, but catheter should be available at all times.

Type of pouch: None; a drainable pouch can be applied if there is leakage of stool between intubations.

Need for irrigation: Occasionally to liquefy thick fecal matter, the pouch can be irrigated with 1 to 1.5 oz of saline or water. Specific care should be clarified by the ET nurse or physician.

BLADDER ASSESSMENT

- If bladder distention is detected during abdominal assessment, a bladder scan can be conducted at the bedside to determine the amount of residual urine.

Ultrasound Bladder Scanner

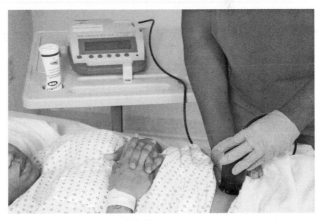

(From Perry AG, et al.: *Clinical nursing skills and techniques,* ed 9, St. Louis, 2018, Elsevier.)

Conditions Affecting Urination

- Food and fluid intake
- Dehydration
- Infection
- Swelling or obstruction
- Kidney diseases
  - Acute or chronic kidney failure

- Calculi
- Cardiac or circulatory disorders
- Tumors
- Muscle tone
- Medication
- Incontinence
  - Functional
  - Reflex
  - Stress
  - Urge
  - Total

URINE CHARACTERISTICS

Characteristics	Normal	Abnormal	Assess for
Amount in 24 hrs	1200 mL	<1200 mL	Renal failure
	1500 mL	>1500 mL	Fluid intake
Color	Straw	Amber	Dehydration, fluid intake
		Light straw	Overhydration
		Orange	Medications
		Red	Blood, injury, medications
Consistency	Clear	Cloudy, thick	Infection
Odor	Faint	Offensive	Infection, medications
Sterile	Yes	Organisms	Infection, poor hygiene
pH	4.5	<4.5	Infection
	8.0	>8.0	Diabetes, starvation, dehydration

Continued

URINE CHARACTERISTICS—Cont'd

Characteristics	Normal	Abnormal	Assess for
Specific gravity	1.010	<1.010	Diabetes insipidus, kidney failure
	1.025	>1.025	Diabetes, underhydration
Glucose	None	Present	Diabetes
Ketones	None	Present	Diabetes, starvation, vomiting
Blood	None	Present	Tumors, injury, kidney disease

TYPES OF COMMON BLADDER OSTOMIES
Urinary Diversion (Ileal Conduit)

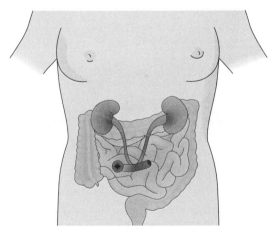

(From Perry AG, et al.: *Clinical nursing skills and techniques,* ed 9, St. Louis, 2018, Elsevier.)

Urinary Diversion (Ileal Conduit)—Cont'd

Drainage characteristics: Urine only. Output is
  constant. Mucus is expelled with urine. Mild odor
  unless there is a urinary tract infection. Urine is
  irritating when in contact with skin. Segment of
  ileum or colon is used to construct stoma.
Skin barrier option: Highly desirable for peristomal
  skin protection.
Pouch option: Pouch necessary at all times.
Type of pouch: Drainable pouch with spout.
Need for irrigation: None.

Continent Urostomy

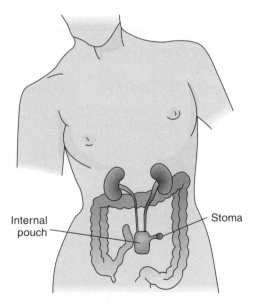

(From Perry AG, et al.: *Clinical nursing skills and techniques,*
ed 9, St. Louis, 2018, Elsevier.)

Continent Urostomy—Cont'd

Drainage characteristics: Urine is maintained in a surgically constructed ileal pouch until emptied by means of a catheter inserted into the stoma. Uses two nipple valves—one to prevent the reflux of urine from backing up into the kidneys and the other to keep urine in the pouch until eliminated. Pouch is drained approximately four times daily. Daily schedule for pouch catheterization should be recommended by the ET nurse or physician.

Skin barrier option: None; an absorbent pad provides peristomal skin protection.

Pouch option: None, but a catheter should be available at all times.

Type of pouch: None; a urostomy pouch can be applied if there is leakage of urine between intubations.

Need for irrigation: Irrigate daily with 1 to 1.5 oz of saline solution and repeat several times as needed until the returns are clear. Specific care should be clarified by the ET nurse or physician.

For additional information on abdominal assessment, consult the following:

Ball JW, et al: *Seidel's guide to physical examination,* ed 9, St. Louis, 2019, Elsevier.

Jarvis C: *Physical examination and health assessment,* ed 8, St. Louis, 2020, Elsevier.

Potter PA, Perry AG, Stockert PA, Hall AM: *Fundamentals of nursing,* ed 10, St. Louis, 2021, Elsevier.

Wilson SF, Giddens JF: *Health assessment for nursing practice,* ed 6, St. Louis, 2017, Elsevier.

Yoost BL, Crawford LR: *Fundamentals of nursing: active learning for collaborative practice,* ed 2, St. Louis, 2020, Elsevier.

CHAPTER 17

Breast and Genital Assessment

BREAST AND GENITAL HEALTH ASSESSMENT QUESTIONS

Breasts: Male and Female

- Have you noticed any changes in the look or feel of your breasts?
- Do you have mammograms done? If so, how often? When was your last mammogram?
- Have you had any nipple discharge or discomfort?
- Do you or any family members have a history of breast cancer?
- Have you ever had surgery on your breasts?

Female Genitals

- When was your last menstrual period? Do you have symptoms associated with your period?
- Have you ever been pregnant? If so, when? Do you have living children? If so, how many?
- Are you sexually active? Do you practice safe sex?
- Do you use contraception?

- Are you having any pain or difficulty associated with intercourse?
- Have you used hormones for contraception or for postmenopausal symptoms?
- Do you drink caffeine or alcohol?
- Have you experienced vaginal discharge, painful lumps, or tissue abrasions or tears in the perineal area, or genital warts or lesions?
- Do you have a family history of endometrial, ovarian, or cervical cancer?

Male Genitals

- Have you noticed any changes in urination flow or frequency? Does your urine have an odor?
- Are you sexually active? Do you practice safe sex?
- Have you had a vasectomy?
- Do you drink caffeine or alcohol?
- Do you have any pain, swelling, or discharge from your penis?
- Have you ever had genital warts on your penis or around your anus?
- Have you noticed any lumps, enlargement, or pain in your testicles?
- Do you do a monthly testicular self-examination?
- Do you have swelling or any protrusion in your groin? If so, does it get worse when you cough or lift heavy objects?
- Do you have difficulty with achieving or maintaining an erection or with the process of ejaculation?

BREAST INSPECTION AND PALPATION

- Assess breasts for symmetry, size, and shape.
  - One breast is often slightly larger than the other.
- Observe breast contour and skin covering the breast tissue.

- Note any lumps, masses, flattening, retraction, or dimpling of the breast tissue.
  - Retraction or dimpling may result from invasion of underlying ligaments and tissues by tumors.
  - Watch for any drainage, bruising, or excoriation.
  - Note the color, venous pattern, and presence of lesions, erythema, dimpling, or inflammation of the skin.
- Nipples can be inverted, everted, or flat and should not have any visible drainage unless the patient is a female who is breastfeeding.
- Use the pads of the first three fingers to compress the breast tissue gently against the chest wall, noting the characteristics of the fleshy tissue, while the patient is lying supine with arms raised behind the head.
  - Consistency of normal breast tissue can vary across the life span, from person to person, and between genders.
- When palpating the nipple and areola, note the consistency of the underlying tissue and any color changes that occur with gentle compression.
- Document the location of any abnormalities using a systematic approach that divides the breast into four quadrants extending into the axillary areas.
- Encourage women and men to be familiar with the appearance and feel of their breasts, reporting any changes immediately.
- Monthly breast self-examination (BSE) is not currently recommended. Clinical breast examinations are recommended every 1 to 3 years for women 29 to 39 years old and annually for women 40 and older.

Breast Quadrants

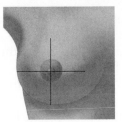

Right breast

(From Yoost BL, Crawford LR: *Fundamentals of nursing: active learning for collaborative practice*, ed 2, St. Louis, 2020, Elsevier.)

EXTERNAL FEMALE GENITALIA

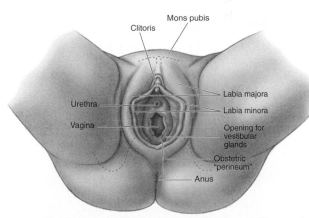

(From Herlihy B: *The human body in health and illness,* ed 6, St. Louis, 2018, Elsevier.)

EXTERNAL FEMALE GENITALIA INSPECTION AND PALPATION

- Apply clean gloves.
- With the patient in the dorsal recumbent position, inspect the outer genitalia for redness, swelling, lesions, masses, or infestations.

- Note the hair growth and distribution in the pelvic area.
- Palpate the inguinal area for presence of lymph nodes.
- Carefully separate and palpate the labia majora and minora from front to back.
  - Inspect the labia, the folds in between, and the clitoris.
  - Note any redness, swelling, lesions, or discharge.
- Note the urethral meatus in relation to the other structures of the perineum.
- Inspect the vaginal orifice for color, smoothness, and moisture.
- Inspect the anus, noting any redness, swelling, or hemorrhoids.
  - Palpate the perianal area for lesions or nodules.

EXTERNAL MALE GENITALIA

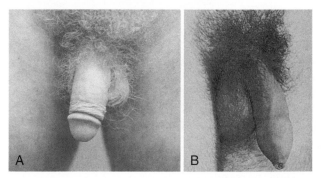

(From Ball JW, Dains JE, Flynn JA, et al.: *Seidel's guide to physical examination,* ed 9, St. Louis, 2019, Elsevier.)

EXTERNAL MALE GENITALIA INSPECTION AND PALPATION

- Apply clean gloves.
- Note the size and shape of the penis and testes as well as the distribution of pubic hair across the perineal area.

- Note whether the penis is circumcised or uncircumcised and whether the foreskin retracts easily.
- Observe for smegma (a whitish substance under the foreskin), abnormal discharge, or lesions.
- Note the appearance of the urethral meatus.
- Carefully pinch the glans between the thumb and index finger to open the urethral meatus for examination.
- Return the foreskin to its original position.
- Palpate the shaft of the penis by compressing the shaft of the penis between the thumb and the first two fingers at incremental intervals from the base to the glans.
  - Note any tenderness or pain response, lesions, scars, swelling, or edema.
- Examine the scrotum for lesions, rashes, edema, tenderness, masses, and potential malignant lesions.
- Palpate the testes one at a time by gently pressing the testes between the thumb and first two fingers, moving from the base to the distal portion in an incremental manner until the entire surface has been examined.
  - Note the size, shape, and symmetry of the organs, as well as any pain or discharge from the penis during testicular palpation.
- Verify the patient's knowledge of testicular self-assessment.

For additional information on breast and genital assessment, consult the following:

Ball JW, et al: *Seidel's guide to physical examination,* ed 9, St. Louis, 2019, Elsevier.

Jarvis C: *Physical examination and health assessment,* ed 8, St. Louis, 2020, Elsevier.

Potter PA, Perry AG, Stockert PA, Hall AM: *Fundamentals of nursing,* ed 10, St. Louis, 2021, Elsevier.

Wilson SF, Giddens JF: *Health assessment for nursing practice,* ed 6, St. Louis, 2017, Elsevier.

Yoost BL, Crawford LR: *Fundamentals of nursing: active learning for collaborative practice,* ed 2, St. Louis, 2020, Elsevier.

CHAPTER 18

Safety

PATIENT SAFETY IN THE HOSPITAL SETTING

- Orient the patient to equipment in the room, including the call light or bell, side rails and bed controls, room and bathroom lights, bathroom location, and safety equipment.
- Leave the bed in the lowest position with the wheels locked when not providing patient care.
- Keep patient rooms free of excess debris and equipment.
- Ensure that electrical cords and wires are not in walking areas.
- Clean up any water or spills from the floor.
- Immediately place used needles and sharps in appropriate sharps containers.
- Never leave medication unattended in a patient room.
- Identify the patient before administering medications or treatments.

- Always follow the Six Rights of Medications Administration.
- Check electrical equipment for proper functioning.
- Wash hands or use hand sanitizer before and after each patient encounter.

LIFE SPAN SAFETY CONSIDERATIONS
Infant, Toddler, and Preschooler
- Use only approved cribs and toys
- Childproof home environment
- Cut food in small pieces
- Fence pool areas
- Never leave unattended
- Use properly installed child safety seats following manufacturer's recommendations

School Age
- Supervise swimming and water activities
- Recommend safety precautions for trampolines and other activities
- Encourage the use of bicycle helmets

Adolescent
- Monitor for depression, drug use, and alcohol use
- Educate regarding safe sexual practices
- Recommend safety courses for motor vehicles
- Limit exposure to violence from television, games, movies, internet
- Encourage the use of bicycle helmets

Adult
- Address workplace concerns, such as stress, working overtime, or being out of work
- Assess for illicit substance and prescription drug use
- Educate regarding the dangers of driving while impaired or distracted
- Discourage unsafe sexual practices

Older Adult
- Assess for fall risks
- Monitor decreased senses and mobility
- Promote medication safety precautions
- Evaluate ability to drive safely

POISON SAFETY
- Poisoning: the intentional or unintentional ingestion, inhalation, injection, or absorption through the skin of any substance that is harmful to the body.
- **The National Poison Control Center phone number in the United States is 1-800-222-1222.**
- Signs and symptoms of poisoning vary depending on the amount of toxin and route of absorption:
  - Some poisons enlarge the pupils, whereas others shrink them.
  - Some result in excessive drooling, whereas others dry the mouth and skin.
  - Some speed the heart, whereas others slow the heart.
  - Some increase the breathing rate, whereas others slow it.
  - Some cause pain, whereas others are painless.
  - Some cause hyperactivity, whereas others cause drowsiness.
- Almost every possible sign or symptom of a poisoning can also be caused by a non–poison related medical problem. A thorough assessment should be completed, and medical attention should be advised.

FIRE SAFETY
- Many health care facilities use the fire emergency response defined by the acronym **RACE:**

- **R:** *Rescue* all patients in immediate danger and move them to safe areas.
- **A:** *Alarm:* Activate the manual-pull station and/or fire alarm and have someone call 911.
- **C:** *Contain* the fire by closing doors, confining the fire, and preventing the spread of smoke.
- **E:** *Extinguish* the fire if possible after all patients are removed from the area.
- Know the facility's fire drill and evacuation plan.
- Close windows and doors.
- Turn off oxygen supply.
- All extinguishers are labeled A, B, C, or D according to the types of fires they are meant to extinguish. Some extinguishers can be used for more than one type of fire and are labeled with more than one letter. The letters correspond to:
  - **A:** paper or wood
  - **B:** liquid or gas
  - **C:** electrical
  - **D:** combustible metal

SEIZURES
Seizure Terminology
- **Absence seizure:** Previously called *petit mal.* Brief lapses in consciousness characterized by brief staring spells.
- **Aura:** A warning of a seizure.
- **Complex partial:** The person is conscious but impaired.
- **Epilepsy:** Recurrent seizures.
- **Febrile seizures:** Generally occur in infants and young children; they are most often generalized tonic-clonic seizures. They typically occur in children with a high fever, usually higher than 102°F.

- **Focal seizure:** Abnormal electrical activity in one area of the brain. May or may not cause loss of consciousness.
- **Generalized seizures:** Widespread abnormal electrical activity of the brain; can be absence or tonic-clonic.
- **Postictal state:** The period after a generalized or focal seizure during which the person usually feels sleepy or confused.
- **Seizure:** Abnormal electrical activity in the brain.
- **Status epilepticus (SE):** A state of continuous or frequently reoccurring seizures lasting 30 minutes or more.
- **Tonic-clonic seizure:** Previously called *grand mal. Tonic* means stiffening, and *clonic* means rhythmic shaking. There is generalized abnormal electrical activity affecting the whole brain.

Care of the Patient with Seizures
- Equipment and procedures
  - Bed should be in the lowest position.
  - Side rails should be *up* and padded.
  - Oxygen and suction equipment should be nearby.
  - Indicate "seizure precautions" on plan of care.
  - Note if patient has an aura before seizures.
  - Always transport the patient with portable oxygen.
  - Patients with frequent generalized tonic-clonic seizures should wear helmets.
- During the seizure
  - Call for help and do NOT try to restrain the person.
  - *STAY WITH THE PERSON* and time the seizure.
  - Help the person to lie down. Place something soft under the head.

- Turn the person on his or her side if possible.
- Remove glasses and loosen tight clothing.
- Do NOT place anything between the teeth.
- Do NOT attempt to remove dentures.
- Monitor the duration of the seizure and the type of movement.
- After the seizure
  - Turn the person to one side to allow saliva to drain; suction if needed.
  - Perform vital signs and neurological checks as needed.
  - Do NOT offer food or drink until the person is fully awake.
  - Reorient the person.
  - Notify physician *unless* the person is being monitored specifically for seizures.
  - Notify physician *immediately* if seizure occurs without regaining consciousness or if an injury occurs.
  - Record all observations.
  - Document the time and length of the seizure and if there was an aura.
  - Document the sequence of behaviors during the seizures (e.g., eye movement).
  - Document any injuries and how they were treated.
  - Note what happened with the person just after the seizure (did he or she reorient?).

SPECIAL PATIENT SITUATIONS
Hospitalized patients with the following problems may require additional safety measures.

Alcohol Withdrawal
- **Signs and symptoms:** Confusion, sweating, pallor, palpitations, hypotension, seizures, coma.

- **Nursing interventions:** Protocols may vary by facility. Withdrawal protocols may include seizure precautions, keeping the side rails up and padded, taking vital signs frequently (every 30 to 60 minutes or per hospital protocol), and close observation. Provide a safe environment. Perform neurological, memory, and orientation checks. Document any withdrawal activity and actions taken.

Bleeding or Hemorrhage
- **Signs and symptoms:** Obvious bleeding, hypotension, tachycardia, tachypnea.
- **Nursing interventions:** Locate the source of the bleeding. Apply direct pressure with sterile gauze. Call for assistance but stay with the patient. Assess for early signs of shock, such as a change in sensorium, and later signs of shock, such as hypotension; pale skin; and a rapid, weak pulse.
- **Prevention:** Closely supervise confused or heavily medicated patients and patients just returning from surgery. Make sure surgical dressings are secure. Encourage patients to call for assistance if bleeding begins. Document any bleeding and actions taken.

Choking
- **Signs and symptoms:** Patient holding throat and anxious, gasping or crowing sound.
- **Nursing interventions:** Follow standard abdominal thrust maneuver guidelines.
- **Prevention:** Closely supervise confused and heavily medicated patients. Make sure patients are sitting up or are placed in high Fowler position when eating. Encourage the use of the call lights. Assess the patient's ability to chew and swallow.

Order a diet appropriate to the patient's eating ability. Document any choking situations and actions taken.

The Confused Patient
- **Signs and symptoms:** Wandering, disoriented to person, place, time, or situation.
- **Nursing interventions:** Assess for the source of the confusion. Possible sources include age, medications, disease, and infection. Confused patients may be at risk for falls. Keep the environment safe by removing unnecessary equipment and wiping up spills immediately. Check on patient often. Place in room near the nurses station.

Drug Reactions
- **Signs and symptoms:** Vary depending on which medication was taken.
- **Nursing interventions:** Assess for difficulty breathing, wheezing, tearing, palpitations, skin rash, pruritus, nausea or vomiting, rhinitis, diarrhea, dilated or constricted pupils, and a change in mood or mental status. These are general drug reactions, not the side effects of specific drugs. Immediately report all drug reactions.
- **Prevention:** Closely supervise confused and heavily medicated patients and patients who are taking medications for the first time. Encourage the use of the call lights if any of the signs of a drug reaction occur. Know your patient's drug allergies. Document all drug reactions and actions taken.

Syncope and Common Causes
- **Neurologic:** transient ischemic attacks, strokes
- **Metabolic:** hypoxia, hyperventilation, hypoglycemia, fluid and electrolyte imbalances

- **Cardiac:** orthostatic hypotension, dysrhythmias, vasovagal reaction
- **Vasomotor:** obstructive lesions, arrhythmias
- **Nursing interventions:** Assess for dizziness, light-headedness, visual blurring or any visual or hearing changes, weakness, apprehension, nausea, sweating, assess vital signs, including blood pressure, and pulse. Stay with the patient. Help the patient sit or lower to the chair, bed, or floor. Protect the patient's head at all times. Call for help. Elevate the legs, assess vital signs, help the patient sit up slowly when he or she is ready, and document the episode per facility policy.

MORSE FALL SCALE ASSESSMENT

Risk Factor	Scale	Score
History of falls	Yes	25
	No	0
Secondary diagnosis	Yes	15
	No	0
Ambulatory aid	Furniture	30
	Crutches/cane/ walker	15
	None/bed rest/ wheelchair/nurse	0
IV/heparin lock	Yes	20
	No	0
Gait/transferring	Impaired	20
	Weak	10
	Normal/bed rest/ immobile	0

Continued

MORSE FALL SCALE ASSESSMENT—Cont'd

Risk Factor	Scale	Score
Mental status	Forgets limitations	15
	Oriented to own ability	0

To obtain the Morse Fall Score add the score from each category.

Morse Fall Score	
High risk	45 and higher
Moderate risk	25-44
Low risk	0-24

From Morse JM, Black C, Oberle K, et al: A prospective study to identify the fall-prone patient, *Soc Sci Med* 28(1):81–86, 1989.

FALL PREVENTION
Fall Prevention at the Hospital
- Frequently observe the at-risk patient.
- Place the patient in a room near the nurses' station.
- Use a low bed.
- Use a mattress or wheelchair seat with pressure alarms.
- Use top side rails. (*Note:* Use of four side rails is considered a restraint.)
- Always return the bed to its lowest position after care.
- Keep the call light within reach of the patient.
  - Remind the patient about how to use the call light.
  - Immediately answer the call light.
- Keep the wheels of any wheeled device (bed, wheelchair) in the locked position.
- Leave lights or a night light on at night depending on the patient's cognitive status and personal preference.

- Keep personal items (tissues, water, urinals) within the patient's reach.
- Frequently orient and reorient the patient.
- If the patient is ambulatory, require the use of nonskid footwear.
- Clear any potential obstructions from the walking areas.
- Ensure that patient clothing fits properly; improper fit can cause tripping.

Fall Assessment Checklist

One or more of the following items can place a person at risk for falls:

- Agitation
- Cardiac disease
- Disorientation or confusion
- Diuretic use
- Language barriers
- Electrolyte imbalance
- Hearing or visual loss
- History of falls
- Hypotension
- Neurological disease
- Age 70 or older
- New medications
- Peripheral vascular disease
- Psychotropic drug use
- Recent cerebrovascular accident
- Recent myocardial infarction
- Uncontrolled diabetes
- Urinary frequency
- Use of a cane or walker
- Weakness

Fall Prevention at Home

Health teaching for patients discharged to or residing in the home needs to include environmental interventions for fall prevention.

- Remove obstacles from walking paths (clutter, throw rugs, and cords).
- Ensure adequate lighting in areas such as bathrooms, halls, and stairways.
- Use nightlights in common areas such as hallways or in walkways to the bathroom.
- Keep assistive devices (canes and walkers) within reach.
- Repair loose or uneven floor/stairway surfaces.
- Install and maintain handrails and grab bars.
- Use devices such as long-handled grabbers rather than reaching or stooping.
- Keep frequently used items close by or within reach.
- If there are children in the house, install gates in doorways and at the top and bottom of stairs.

RESTRAINTS
When to Use Restraints
- To prevent injury
- To restrict movement
- To immobilize a body part
- To prevent harm to self or others
- Restraints should be used only when all other methods of keeping a patient safe have been tried.
- Know the organizational policy regarding the use of restraints.

Types of Restraints
- Jackets or vests, belts, mittens, wrist or ankle, crib net, elbow

Guidelines
- Obtain physician's order and follow facility protocol.
- Explain purpose to patient; check circulation every 30 minutes.
- Release temporarily (once per hour).
- Provide range of motion.

- Document need and assessment schedule.
- Report problems and tolerance; provide emotional support.
- Never secure restraints to the side rails or the nonstationary portion of the main frame of the bed. Tie the restraint to a portion of the bed frame that moves with the patient.
- Frequent checks of the patient under restraint are essential because injuries due to entrapment and death from strangulation or asphyxiation are most likely to result when the patient attempts to escape physical restraint.

Complications
- Skin breakdown (pad bony areas).
- Nerve damage (do not overtighten; release often).
- Circulatory impairment (check for problems often; provide range of motion).
- Death (from inadequate monitoring or improper use).

Prevention
- Keep the top side rails up when you are not with the patient.
- Monitor vital signs and the patient's drug doses and levels.
- Monitor the patient's electrolytes and neurological status.
- Reorient patient to place and time as needed.
- Place call light in easy reach.
- Attend closely to personal care needs.
- Encourage family, friends, and clergy to visit often.

How to Tie a Quick-Release Restraint Tie
- Never tie a restraint in a knot, because the knot could prohibit quick exit in the event of an emergency requiring evacuation. Instead, use quick-release ties or mechanisms such as buckles.

Quick-release restraint tie

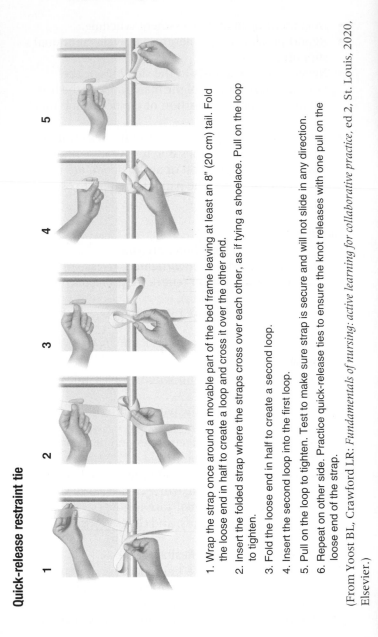

1. Wrap the strap once around a movable part of the bed frame leaving at least an 8" (20 cm) tail. Fold the loose end in half to create a loop and cross it over the other end.
2. Insert the folded strap where the straps cross over each other, as if tying a shoelace. Pull on the loop to tighten.
3. Fold the loose end in half to create a second loop.
4. Insert the second loop into the first loop.
5. Pull on the loop to tighten. Test to make sure strap is secure and will not slide in any direction.
6. Repeat on other side. Practice quick-release ties to ensure the knot releases with one pull on the loose end of the strap.

(From Yoost BL, Crawford LR: *Fundamentals of nursing: active learning for collaborative practice*, ed 2, St. Louis, 2020, Elsevier.)

HOME SAFETY ASSESSMENT

Health history and physical assessment should dictate specific safety questions, such as the following:

- **Activities of daily living:** Do you require assistance with any of the following: walking, toileting, bathing, dressing, grooming, eating, cooking, driving, shopping, or cleaning?
- **Medications:** Do you know how and when to take your medications? Do you know why you take them? Do you take your medications consistently? Have you been experiencing any side effects? If yes, describe them. Where are your medications stored? Are they out of reach of children, or do they have childproof caps? Are any medications expired?
- **Health issues:** Do you have any injuries or health issues that place you at risk for falling or for drowsiness? Have you ever had a seizure?
- **Safety issues:** Do you have any safety concerns? Do you have a history of falling? Do you have worries about what you would do in case of a fire? Are you stressed out or tired?
- **Chemicals:** How do you store your household chemicals? Are they out of reach of children and pets?
- **Carbon monoxide:** Do you have a carbon monoxide detector in your home?
- **Electrical:** Do you have adequate outlets for all of your appliances and electronic devices? If there are children in the home, are all outlets in your home covered? Do you check for frays or loose wires on electrical cords, including those of electronic devices such as laptops and cell phones? Are your circuit breaker boxes in working order? Are household appliances, such as irons, hair dryers, and electric razors, used away from sources of water? Are the electrical outlets grounded?

- **Fire:** Do you have smoke detectors? A fire extinguisher? An evacuation plan in case of a fire? Do you smoke, or does anyone in your home smoke? How do you heat your home? Is it adequate? Do you use space heaters? Do you have air-conditioning? Fans?
- **Needles:** Do you use hypodermic needles? How do you dispose of them?

For additional information on safety, consult the following:

Ignatavicius DD, Workman ML, Rebar CR: *Medical-surgical nursing: patient-centered collaborative care,* ed 9, St. Louis, 2018, Elsevier.

Lewis SL, Bucher L, Heitkemper MM, et al: *Medical-surgical nursing,* ed 10, St. Louis, 2017, Elsevier.

Potter PA, Perry AG, Stockert PA, Hall AM: *Fundamentals of nursing,* ed 10, St. Louis, 2021, Elsevier.

Yoost BL, Crawford LR: *Fundamentals of nursing: active learning for collaborative practice,* ed 2, St. Louis, 2020, Elsevier.

CHAPTER 19

Equivalents and Dosage Calculation

EQUIVALENT MEASURES

Metric System

To change from a larger to a smaller unit, MULTIPLY the number by 10, 100, and so on or move the decimal point to the RIGHT. To change from a smaller to larger unit, DIVIDE the number by 10, 100, and so on or move the decimal to the LEFT.

- Weight
  - 1 kilogram (kg/Kg) = 1000 grams (g)
  - 1 gram (Gm/gm/g/G) = 1000 milligrams (mg)
  - 1 milligram (mg) = 1000 micrograms (mcg)
- Volume
  - 1 liter (L) = 1000 milliliters (mL)
  - 1 deciliter (dL) = 100 milliliters (mL)
  - 1 milliliter (mL) = 1 cubic centimeter (cc)
- Length
  - 1 meter (m) = 100 centimeters (cm)
  - 1 meter (m) = 1000 millimeters (mm)
  - 1 centimeter (cm) = 10 millimeters (mm)

Apothecary System

- Old system, no longer used on drug labels
- Basic measures
  - Weight: grains (gr)
  - Volume: minims (m), drams (dr), ounces (oz)
- Metric-to-apothecary conversions
  - Grams to grains: Multiply grams (g) by 15
  - Milligrams to grains: Divide milligrams (mg) by 60
- Apothecary-to-metric conversions
  - Grains to grams: Divide grains (gr) by 15
  - Grains to milligrams: Multiply grains (gr) by 60

Household System

- Weight
  - 1 pound (lb) = 16 ounces (oz)
- Volume
  - 1 tablespoon (tbsp/T) = 3 teaspoons (tsp/t)
  - 1 cup (c) = 16 tablespoons (tbsp/T) = 8 ounces
  - 2 cups = 1 pint (pt)
  - 2 pints (pt) = 1 quart (qt)
  - 4 quarts (qt) = 1 gallon (gal)
- Kilogram-to-pound conversions
  - 1 kilogram (kg) = 2.2 pounds (lb)
  - Kilograms to pounds: Multiply kilograms by 2.2
  - Pounds to kilograms: Divide pounds by 2.2
- Centimeter-to-inches conversions
  - 2.54 cm = 1 inch (in)
  - Inches to centimeters (cm): Multiply inches by 2.54
  - Centimeter to inches: Divide centimeters by 2.54
- Common household-to-metric conversions
  - 15 drops (gtt) = 1 mL
  - 1 tsp/t = 5ml
  - 1 tbsp/T = 15 mL
  - 1 ounce = 30 mL
  - 1 cup/c = 240 mL

- 1 pint/pt = 480 mL
- 1 quart/qt = 960 mL or ~1 L
- 1 gallon/gal = 3785 mL or ~4 L

DOSAGE CALCULATIONS
- Always think logically and critically when calculating dosages.
- Estimate the answer before doing the calculation.
- Double-check the math in all dosage calculations.

Methods of Dosage Calculation
- Dimensional analysis
  - Removes the need for multiple-step calculations
  - Provides a consistent method for calculating medication dosages
  - Can be used in all situations
    - Basic calculations
    - Determining pediatric doses
    - Calculating titration of potent drugs in critical care units
- Begin by identifying the units of measure (e.g., mg, capsule) needed for the answer to the problem.
- The unit used in the answer must have the same unit as the numerator, or top of the equation, and the denominator, or bottom of the equation.
- Start the equation with the dose to be given, then the concentration or supply available.
- For example, the prescribed medication is "amoxicillin 0.5 g po every 8 hours," and the available quantity is amoxicillin 250 mg per 1 capsule.
- A unit conversion is needed from grams to milligrams.
- Notice that *capsule* must be in the numerator in the problem, because it is the unit needed in the

answer; the nurse needs to figure out how many capsules to administer per dose.

$$\frac{0.5\,g}{1\,dose} \times \frac{1\,capsule}{250\,mg} \times \frac{1000\,mg}{1\,g} =$$

In dimensional analysis, the first step is to cross off units that appear in both the numerator and denominator:

$$\frac{0.5\,\cancel{g}}{1\,dose} \times \frac{1\,capsule}{250\,\cancel{mg}} \times \frac{1000\,\cancel{mg}}{1\,\cancel{g}} =$$

- After the units occurring in both numerator and denominator are crossed off, the only units left in the equation are the correct ones for the answer to the nurse's question.
- Next, the numbers on the top of the equation are multiplied, and the numbers on the bottom are multiplied. The final step is to divide the numerator by the denominator and add the correct units to the numeric answer:

$$\frac{500\,capsules}{250\,doses} = \frac{2\,capsules}{1\,dose}$$

Ratio and Proportion
- Ratio is the relationship between two numbers 1:2 or 1/2.
- Proportion is the comparison of two ratios 1:2 = 2:4 or 1/2 = 2/4.
- If three of the four numbers of a proportion are known, the fourth can be easily calculated 1/2 = x/4; x = 2.
- In dosage calculations, set up the proportions using the same labels in the numerator and the denominator.

- Conversions must be completed before setting up the proportions (i.e., grams to milligrams or micrograms to grams, etc.).
- Example: "amoxicillin 500 mg po every 8 hours" and the available supply is amoxicillin 400 mg per 5 mL.
- How many mL will be administered with each dose?
- Set up the proportion with the available supply and the ordered dose:

$$\frac{400\,\text{mg}}{5\,\text{mL}} = \frac{500\,\text{mg}}{\text{x}\,\text{mL}}$$

- Cross multiply (multiply the numerator on one side of the = times the denominator on the other):

$$400\text{x} = 2500$$

- Solve for x by dividing both sides by 400. Add the units needed for the answer, in this case mL:

$$\frac{400\text{x}}{400} = \frac{2500}{400} = 6.25\,\text{mL}$$

Formula
- Formula must be memorized.
- Conversions must be completed before setting up the formula (i.e., grams to milligrams or micrograms to grams, etc.)
- Formula:

$$\frac{\text{Dose ordered (D)}}{\text{Dose on hand (H)}} \times \text{amount or quantity on hand (Q)}$$

$$= \text{unknown or amount to administer (x)}$$

$$\text{or } \frac{\text{D}}{\text{H}} \times \text{Q} = \text{x}$$

- Example: "amoxicillin 500 mg every 8 hours," and the available supply is amoxicillin 400 mg per 5 mL.

$$\frac{500\,\text{mg}}{400\,\text{mg}} \times 5\,\text{mL} = 6.25\,\text{mL}$$

INTRAVENOUS (IV) CALCULATIONS

- Calculating the rate on a volumetric IV pump
  - Most IVs are run on volumetric pumps.
  - When a volume of fluid is ordered to run over a certain amount of time, the nurse must figure out what rate to set on the pump.
  - Order: 1000 mL 0.9% Normal Saline to run over 8 hours. How many mL per hour will be set to run on the IV pump?

$$\frac{1000\,\text{mL}}{8\,\text{hr}} = \frac{125\,\text{mL}}{\text{hr}}$$

- IV drip rates without an IV pump
  - When an IV pump is not available, the nurse calculates how many drops per minute of fluid should infuse.
  - To determine the drops per minute, the nurse must know the IV tubing type and drop factor.
  - 2 types of IV tubing: macrodrip and microdrip, with different drop factors (number of drops to make 1 mL).
  - Macrodrip tubing has a drop factor of 10 drops (gtt) per mL, 15 drops per mL, or 20 drops per mL (marked on the tubing package).
  - Microdrip tubing has a drop factor of 60 drops per mL.
  - If the amount of IV fluid to be infused per hour is known, hours are converted into minutes.

- Order: 125 mL/hr. Tubing size: macrodrip tubing, 15 drops per mL. Using dimensional analysis:

$$\frac{125\,\text{mL}}{1\,\text{hr}} \times \frac{15\,\text{gtts}}{1\,\text{mL}} \times \frac{1\,\text{hr}}{60\,\text{min}} = \frac{31.25\,\text{gtt}}{\text{min}} \text{ or } \frac{\sim 31\,\text{gtt}}{\text{min}}$$

- The nurse counts the number of drops dripping into the chamber in 1 minute and regulates the IV accordingly.

- Order: 125 mL/hr. Tubing size: microdrip tubing, 60 drops per mL. Using dimensional analysis:

$$\frac{125\,\text{mL}}{1\,\text{hr}} \times \frac{60\,\text{gtts}}{1\,\text{mL}} \times \frac{1\,\text{hr}}{60\,\text{min}} = \frac{125\,\text{gtt}}{\text{min}}$$

- The nurse counts the number of drops dripping into the chamber in 1 minute and regulates the IV accordingly.

For additional information on equivalents and dosage calculations, consult the following:

Burcham JR, Rosenthal LD: *Lehne's pharmacology for nursing care,* ed 9, St. Louis, 2016, Elsevier.

Clayton BC, Willihnganz M: *Basic pharmacology for nurses,* ed 17, St. Louis, 2017, Elsevier.

Gray Morris D: *Calculate with confidence,* ed 7, St. Louis, 2018, Elsevier.

Mulholland JM: *The nurse, the math, the meds: drug calculations using dimensional analysis,* ed 4, St. Louis, 2019, Elsevier.

Potter PA, Perry AG, Stockert PA, Hall AM: *Fundamentals of nursing*, ed 10, St. Louis, 2021, Elsevier.

Skidmore-Roth L: *Mosby's 2019 nursing drug reference,* ed 32, St. Louis, 2019, Elsevier.

Workman ML, LaCharity L: *Understanding pharmacology: essentials for medication safety,* ed 2, St. Louis, 2016, Elsevier.

Yoost BL, Crawford LR: *Fundamentals of nursing: active learning for collaborative practice*, ed 2, St. Louis, 2020, Elsevier.

CHAPTER 20

Medication Administration

MEDICATION TERMINOLOGY

- **Absorption:** The passage of drug molecules into the blood.
- **Allergic reaction:** An unpredictable response to a drug.
- **Duration:** Length of time in the body.
- **Half-life:** Time of elimination from body.
- **Interactions:** When one drug modifies the actions of another.
- **Onset:** First response of drug in the body.
- **Peak:** Highest level of drug in the body.
- **Side effects:** Unintended secondary effects.
- **Therapeutic range:** Range at which the level of drug is most beneficial.
- **Trough:** Lowest level of drug in the body.

CONTROLLED SUBSTANCES
- **Schedule I:** Highest potential for abuse: heroin, LSD, marijuana.
- **Schedule II:** High potential for abuse: morphine, cocaine, methadone, and methamphetamine.
- **Schedule III:** Potential for abuse: anabolic steroids, narcotics such as codeine or hydrocodone with aspirin or acetaminophen, and some barbiturates.
- **Schedule IV:** Low potential for abuse: pentazocine, meprobamate, diazepam, and alprazolam.
- **Schedule V:** Lowest potential for abuse: over-the-counter cough medicines with codeine.

MEDICATION ADMINISTRATION SAFETY
Six Rights of Medication Administration
- The right drug
- The right dose
- The right time
- The right route
- The right patient
- The right documentation

Additional Checks before Medication Administration
- Check prescriber order
- Check patient allergies
- Check medication expiration date

Other Medication Administration Safety Information
- Prepare medications in a no-interruption zone.
- Learn about the medications being administered.

- Double-check all calculations.
- Never administer medication that you did not prepare.
- Medication administration cannot be delegated, even to other professionals.
- Unlicensed assistive personnel (UAP) may not administer medications unless they are in a state that allows designation of certified medication technicians in certain facilities. Check with the state's nurse practice act and the facility's policies and procedures.
- If a medication technician or LPN/LVN administers medications, the task is not being delegated; the other staff member is assuming responsibility.
- If there is any question regarding the medication order by the nurse or the patient, do not administer the medication. Contact the primary care provider or pharmacist for clarification.
- Never leave the medication unattended at the bedside.

COMMON ALLERGIC REACTIONS TO MEDICATIONS
- Difficulty breathing
- Palpitations
- Skin rashes
- Nausea
- Vomiting
- Pruritus
- Rhinitis
- Watery eyes
- Wheezing
- Vomiting
- Diarrhea

ROUTES OF ADMINISTRATION

- Oral (PO): by mouth
- Sublingual (SL): under the tongue
- Buccal (B): against the cheek
- Topical: on the skin or mucous membranes
  - Transdermal (TD): on the skin
  - Rectal (PR): in the rectum
  - Otic: in the ear
  - Ophthalmic: in the eye
  - Vaginal: in the vagina
  - Nasal: in the nose
- Parenteral: by injection or infusion
  - Subcutaneous (subcut)
  - Intradermal (ID)
  - Intramuscular (IM)
  - Intravenous (IV)
- Inhalation

INJECTION INFORMATION
Syringes and Needle Sizes

Parenteral Route	Syringe Selection	Needle Selection	Site Selection
Subcutaneous	$^1/_2$-3 mL or Insulin syringe: U-100, U-50, or U-30	25-31 gauge, $^3/_8$-$^5/_8$ inch (up to 1 inch for an obese patient) Preattached to insulin syringe: 29-33 gauge, $^1/_8$-$^5/_{16}$ inch (4-8 mm)*	Abdomen, lateral aspects of the upper arm and thigh, scapular area of the back, and upper ventrodorsal gluteal area
Intradermal	1 mL tuberculin syringe	Preattached 25-27 gauge, $^1/_4$-$^5/_8$ inch	Inner forearm, upper arm, and across the scapula

Continued

INJECTION INFORMATION—Cont'd

Parenteral Route	Syringe Selection	Needle Selection	Site Selection
Intramuscular	Adults: up to 5 mL, depending on site† Infants, small children: 0.5-1 mL	19-25 gauge, 1-3 inch (adult) 22-25 gauge, $5/8$ to 1 inch (pediatric) Oil-based solutions: 18-20 gauge	Ventrogluteal, vastus lateralis, and deltoid Age of patient and corresponding site†: Infant: vastus lateralis Children: vastus lateralis or deltoid Adult: ventrogluteal or deltoid
Intravenous	Depends on amount of medication to be infused	Typically, a large-gauge, 1-inch needle; needleless, blunt-tip cannula, or Luer-Lok used with associated intravenous ports. (Do not use needles in a needleless system to access IV ports.)	Vein

*From Worldwide Injection Technique Questionnaire Study: Mayo Clinic proceedings, 91(9):1212–1223, 2016.

†From Ogston-Tuck S: Intramuscular injection technique: An evidence-based approach. *Nurs Stan*, 29(4):52–59, 2014.

From Yoost BL, Crawford LR: *Fundamentals of nursing: active learning for collaborative practice*, ed 2, St. Louis, 2020, Elsevier.

Angles of Insertion

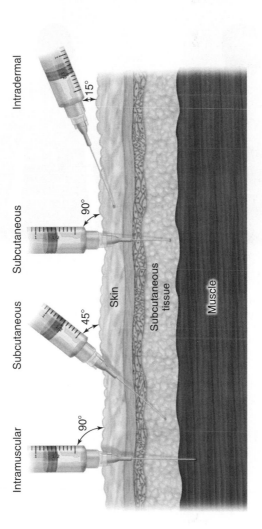

Insertion angles for parenteral injections. (From Yoost BL, Crawford LR: *Fundamentals of nursing: Active learning for collaborative practice,* ed 2, St. Louis, 2020, Elsevier.)

Subcutaneous Injection Sites

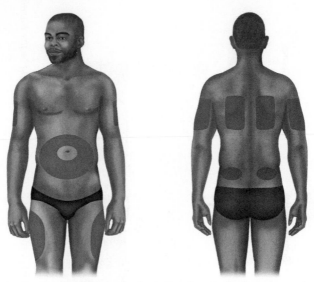

(From Yoost BL, Crawford LR: *Fundamentals of nursing: active learning for collaborative practice*, ed 2, St. Louis, 2020, Elsevier.)

Intramuscular Injection Sites

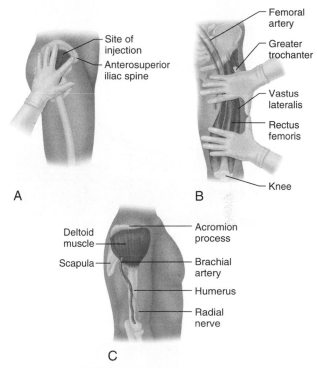

Intramuscular injection sites. (**A**) Ventrogluteal. (**B**) Vastus lateralis. (**C**) Deltoid. (From Yoost BL, Crawford LR: *Fundamentals of nursing: active learning for collaborative practice*, ed 2, St. Louis, 2020, Elsevier.)

Z-track

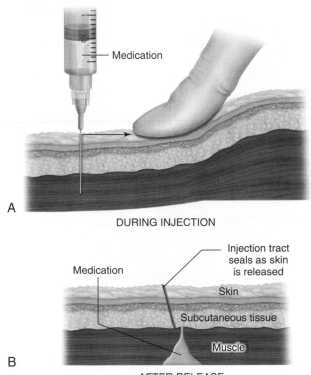

DURING INJECTION

AFTER RELEASE

Z-track intramuscular injection technique: (**A**) During injection. (**B**) After release. (From Yoost BL, Crawford LR: *Fundamentals of nursing: active learning for collaborative practice*, ed 2, St. Louis, 2020, Elsevier.)

INTRAVENOUS INFUSIONS
IV Types
- Peripheral
  - Inserted in a peripheral vein, usually of the hand or arm.
  - Used for administering IV fluid replacement or medications.
  - If an intermittent infusion device (saline lock or PRN adapter) is used, flush with 2 to 3 mL of normal saline before and after each use or at every shift.
- Peripherally inserted central catheter (PICC)
  - A central venous catheter (CVC) inserted in the cephalic or basilic vein or antecubital space and threaded up until it rests in the superior vena cava outside the right atrium.
  - Intermediate to long-term IV therapy.
  - Flush all lumens with 10 mL of preservative-free sterile saline daily or before and after each use.
- Implanted port
  - A CVC device placed surgically under the skin in the upper chest.
  - Long-term intravenous access, usually for oncology or hematology patients.
  - Should be accessed at least monthly and flushed with 10 mL of the prescribed flush, either heparin or saline.
- Triple lumen catheter
  - A CVC device usually inserted into the subclavian vein.
  - Three separate lumens or tubes within the catheter for administering different substances.
  - Flush all lumens with 10 mL of preservative-free sterile saline daily or before and after each use.

Note: Check facility policy and provider orders for specific information on frequency of flushing as well as the amount and type of fluid to use for flushing IV lines.

Common IV solutions

IV Solution	Nursing Considerations
Hypotonic	
0.33% NS	Provides sodium, chloride, and free water. Allows kidneys to select amount of electrolyte to retain or excrete.
0.45% NS	Fluid replacement for clients who do not need extra glucose (diabetics). Useful for establishing renal function. Not used as NaCl replacement therapy. Use cautiously as may cause cardiovascular collapse or increased intracranial pressure.
Isotonic	
D$_5$W	Considered isotonic but becomes free water after dextrose is metabolized, then acts as a hypotonic solution. Because it does not contain sodium, continued use can lead to hyponatremia. Useful in IV medication administration. Can cause hyperglycemia.
0.9% NS	Replaces losses without altering fluid concentrations. Commonly used to reestablish normal extracellular fluid levels in patients with hypovolemia. Helps with NaCl replacement but continued use can lead to hypernatremia/hyperchloremia. Do not use in patients with heart failure, edema, or hypernatremia.

Continued

COMMON IV SOLUTIONS—Cont'd

IV Solution	Nursing Considerations
D$_5$ 0.2% NS	Useful for maintenance of fluids when less sodium is required. The dextrose provides approximately 170 cal/L.
Lactated Ringer	Most closely resembles blood plasma. Contains sodium, potassium, calcium, chloride, and lactate. Used when there is loss of fluid and electrolytes, as in burns, severe diarrhea, or during surgery. Do not use in patients with renal or liver disease.
Hypertonic	
D$_5$ 0.45% NS	Commonly used to treat hypovolemia and maintain normal fluid balance, especially in the postoperative period.
D$_5$ 0.9% NS	Used as replacement fluid. Provides calories, sodium, and chloride. Prolonged use can lead to hypernatremia. Do not use in patients with cardiac or renal failure. Monitor for fluid volume overload.
D$_5$ LR	Same content as lactated Ringer solution but adds calories with the dextrose. Useful when patient's caloric intake is reduced. Monitor for fluid volume overload.
3% NS	Used to treat severe hyponatremia. Administered in an intensive care setting where the patient can be closely monitored.

D$_5$, 5% dextrose; *NS*, normal saline; *W*, water.

From Yoost BL, Crawford LR: *Fundamentals of nursing: active learning for collaborative practice*, ed 2, St. Louis, 2020, Elsevier.

BLOOD ADMINISTRATION

Administering Blood to a Patient

- Blood products are administered to replace lost blood or blood components.
- Blood typing and cross-matching:
  - Typing: Selecting the ABO blood type and Rh antigen factor of a person's blood (other antigens can also affect transfusion compatibility).
  - Cross-matching: Mixing the recipient's serum with the donor's red blood cells in a saline solution; if no agglutination occurs, the blood may be safely given.
- Check facility's policy on infusing blood products.
- Check the patient's ID band for proper identification.
- Check the patient's blood type and Rh antigen.
- Get prescribed blood from blood bank only when ready to infuse.
- Compare the type of blood or blood product ordered with the blood product and the patient's blood type.
- Two nurses should check and cosign blood.
- Start infusion of blood with normal saline solution.
- Administer blood at a slower rate for the first 15 minutes. Blood should be infused within 4 hours.
- Use appropriate blood tubing and needles (may vary per facility).
- Instruct patient to report *any* discomfort (blood reactions).
- Special vital signs are needed (may vary per facility).
- Some facilities may medicate the patient with acetaminophen or diphenhydramine (Benadryl) before infusion.

- Document the times, procedure, vital signs, and patient responses in the electronic health record (EHR).

Blood Reactions

- Possible reactions include difficulty breathing, wheezing, dyspnea, tachypnea, flushing, fever, chills, nausea tachycardia, change in blood pressure, chest pain, disorientation, itching, rash, or hives.
- *If a reaction begins, stop the infusion.* Change the tubing. Begin a normal saline IV and administer prescribed antihistamines.
- Notify the primary care practitioner (PCP), recheck blood, retype, and cross-match. Do *not* discard the blood—the laboratory may want to analyze it for the cause of the reaction.

Blood Type Compatibility

Blood Type	Can Generally Donate to	Can Generally Receive from
A–	A–, A+	A–, O–
B–	B–, B+	B–, O–
AB–	AB–, AB+	AB–, A–, B–, O
A+	A+	A+, A–, O+, O–
B+	B+	B+, B–, O+, O–
AB+	AB+	All blood types
O–	All blood types	O–
O+	O+, A+, B+, AB+	O+, O–

DRUG IN SYRINGE COMPATIBILITY

	Atropine	Buprenorphine	Butorphanol	Chlorpromazine	Codeine	Diazepam	Dimenhydrinate	Diphenhydramine	Droperidol	Fentanyl	Glycopyrrolate	Heparin
Atropine	■		C	C		I	C	C	C	C	C	
Buprenorphine		■										
Butorphanol	C		■	C		I	I	C	C	C		
Chlorpromazine	C		C	■		I	I	C	C	C	C	C
Codeine					■	I						
Diazepam	I		I	I	I	■	I	I	I	I	I	
Dimenhydrinate	C		I	I		I	■	C	C	C	I	
Diphenhydramine	C		C	C		I	C	■	C	C	C	
Droperidol	C		C	C		I	C	C	■	C	C	I
Fentanyl	C		C	C		I	C	C	C	■	C	
Glycopyrrolate	C			C		I	I	C	C	C	■	
Heparin			I	C		I			I			■
Hydroxyzine	C		C	C		I	I	C	C	C	C	
Meperidine	C		C	C		I	C	C	C	C	C	I
Metoclopramide	C		C	C		I	C	C	C	C		
Midazolam	C		C	C		I	C	C	C	C		
Morphine	C		C	C		I	C	C	C	C	C	I
Nalbuphine	C					I			C			
Pentazocine	C		C	C		I	C	C	C	C	I	I
Pentobarbital	C		I	I	I	I	I	I	I	I		
Perphenazine	C		C	C		I	C	C	C	C		
Prochlorperazine	C		C	C		I	I	C	C	C	C	
Promazine	C			C		I	I	C	C	C	C	
Promethazine	C		C	C		I	I	C	C	C	C	
Ranitidine	C			C			C	C		C	C	
Scopolamine Hbr	C		C	C		I	C	C	C	C	C	
Secobarbital	I		I	I	I	I	I	I	I	I		
Thiethylperazine			C			I						

Developed by Providence Memorial Hospital, El Paso, Texas.
NOTE: Give within 15 minutes of mixing.
C = compatible; I = incompatible; ☐ = no documented information.
* = compatibility depends on manufacturer, Wyeth and DuPont forms are incompatible.

	Hydroxyzine	Meperidine	Metoclopramide	Midazolam	Morphine	Nalbuphine	Pentazocine	Pentobarbital	Perphenazine	Prochlorperazine	Promazine	Promethazine	Ranitidine	Scopolamine HBr	Secobarbital	Thiethylperazine
Hydroxyzine	■	C	C	C	C	C	C	C	C	C	C	C	C	C	C	I
Meperidine	C	■	C	C	C	C		C	I	C	C		C		C	I
Metoclopramide	C	C	■	C	C	C		C	I	C	C	C	C	C	C	I
Midazolam				■					I							I
Morphine	I	I	I		■	I	I	I	I	I	I	I	I		I	I
Nalbuphine	I	C	C	I	C	■	C	I	C	I	I	I	C	C	I	
Pentazocine	C	C	C	C	C	C	■	C	I	C	C	C	C	C	C	I
Pentobarbital	C	C	C		C	C	C	■	I	C	C	C	C		C	I
Perphenazine	C	C	C		C		C	I	■	C	C	C	C	C	C	I
Prochlorperazine	C	C			C		I	I		■	C	C	C	C	C	I
Promazine		I			I		I				■		I			
Promethazine	C	C		C	C	C	I		C	C	■	C	C	I	C	I
Ranitidine	C		C		I		C	I	C	C	C	■	C	C	C	I
Scopolamine HBr	C	C		C		C		C	C	C	C	C	■	C		C
Secobarbital	C		C		C	C		I	I	I	C	C	I	■	C	
Thiethylperazine	C		C		■		C	I	C	C	C	C	C	C		■

Parenteral compatibility occurs when two or more drugs are successfully mixed without liquefaction, deliquescence, or precipitation.

From Skidmore-Roth L: *Mosby's 2019 nursing drug reference* 32e, St. Louis, 2019, Elsevier.

For additional information on medication administration,
consult the following:

Burcham JR, Rosenthal LD: *Lehne's pharmacology for nursing care,* ed 9,
    St. Louis, 2016, Elsevier.

Clayton BC, Willihnganz M: *Basic pharmacology for nurses,* ed 17, St. Louis,
    2017, Elsevier.

Gray Morris D: *Calculate with confidence,* ed 7, St. Louis, 2018, Elsevier.

Infusion Nurses Society (INS)*Policies and procedures for infusion nursing*, ed
    5, Norwood, Mass, 2016, Infusion Nurses Society.

Mulholland JM: *The nurse, the math, the meds: drug calculations using
    dimensional analysis,* ed 4, St. Louis, 2019, Elsevier.

Potter PA, Perry AG, Stockert PA, Hall AM: *Fundamentals of nursing*, ed 10,
    St. Louis, 2021, Elsevier.

Skidmore-Roth L: *Mosby's 2019 nursing drug reference,* ed 32, St. Louis,
    2019, Elsevier.

Workman ML, et al: *Understanding pharmacology: essentials for medication
    safety,* ed 2, St. Louis, 2016, Elsevier.

Yoost BL, Crawford LR: *Fundamentals of nursing: active learning for collab-
    orative practice*, ed 2, St. Louis, 2021, Elsevier.

CHAPTER 21

Infection Control

HAND HYGIENE
Guidelines
- Hand hygiene breaks the chain of infection by interrupting the mode of transmission.
- Perform hand hygiene:
  - before and after patient contact or contact with objects that are soiled
  - after removing gloves
  - before eating and after using the bathroom
- Keep fingernails trimmed short.
- Remove artificial nails.
- Remove all jewelry. A plain wedding band is acceptable except when doing a surgical scrub.
- Cover any open sores on hands after washing and wear gloves for patient care.
- Gloves should not be applied to damp hands.
- Educate patients and their visitors in hand hygiene techniques.

Handwashing with Soap and Water
- Perform handwashing when hands are visibly dirty or contaminated;

- when caring for a patient with *Clostridium difficile* (C. diff) or vancomycin-resistant enterococci (VRE);
- before donning sterile gloves or performing a sterile procedure, before meals, and after using the bathroom;
- follow appropriate handwashing guidelines.

Hand Sanitizer
- May be used before and after patient care if soap and water washing is not required.
- Apply hand sanitizer to the palm of one hand. Rub it into the front and back of each hand, between the fingers, and up the wrists. Continue to rub until the sanitizer is dry.

Surgical Hand Scrub
- Reduces the number of pathogens and prevents the spread of microorganisms.
- Performed before surgical procedures with an antiseptic agent.
- Required for all personnel who will be sterile or scrubbed in the surgical suite.
- Remove all jewelry.
- A disposable sponge is used to scrub hands, fingers, and wrists.
- A nail pick is used to clean under fingernails.
- Follow appropriate surgical scrub guidelines.

PERSONAL PROTECTIVE EQUIPMENT
General Information
- Personal protective equipment (PPE) helps prevent the spread of microorganisms between the patient and the caregiver.
- Staff and visitors should be educated in the use of PPE.
- Removal of PPE is done in order of the most contaminated to the least contaminated. Gloves are

removed first because they are considered the most contaminated. Masks are removed last because they protect from particles in the air during the removal of other PPE.

Gloves
- Clean, nonsterile gloves are used when contact with blood and body fluids is possible and for care of patients in contact isolation.
- Sterile gloves are used during sterile procedures such as urinary catheterization.
- Gloves decrease the risk of transferring organisms between patients and caregivers.
- Gloves are removed after patient care, and hands are washed before leaving the room or caring for another patient.

Masks
- Masks protect against infections that travel through the air as larger droplets.
- Masks should be changed if they become wet.
- Special N95 respirator masks protect against diseases that are airborne as smaller droplets.
- N95 masks must be specially fitted.

Gowns
- Waterproof gowns are worn when the caregiver's clothing is likely to come in contact with blood or body fluids, or when caring for a patient in contact isolation.
- Gowns should be changed if they become wet or soiled.
- Disposable gowns are used only once then discarded in the appropriate receptacle.
- Reusable gowns are used only once, then placed in the appropriate laundry bin.

Eye Protection
- Eye protections should be worn if there is a possibility of blood or body fluid splattering onto the caregiver's face. For example, when irrigating a wound, some fluid may splash out of the wound.
- Some masks have shields that protect the eyes.
- Goggles are worn if splatter is likely and the mask does not have a shield.

Caps
- Caps are worn if there is a possibility of blood or body fluid splattering onto the caregiver's head. For example, when irrigating a wound, some fluid may splash out of the wound.
- Caps are worn during some sterile procedures and in the surgical suite to cover the caregiver's and patient's hair. This prevents particles in the hair and on the scalp from contaminating the sterile field.

Shoe Coverings
- Covers are worn to protect shoes from blood and body fluids.
- Operating room personnel should have shoes that are worn only within the surgical suite because street shoes can increase contaminants on the floor.

PRECAUTIONS
Educate patients and their families about precautions being used.

Centers for Disease Control and Prevention Isolation Guidelines
Standard Precautions (Tier One) for Use with All Patients
- Standard precautions apply to blood, blood products, all body fluids, secretions, excretions

(except sweat), nonintact skin, and mucous membranes.

- Perform hand hygiene before, after, and between direct contact with patients. (Examples of between-contact activities are cleaning hands after a patient care activity, moving to a non–patient care activity, and cleaning hands again before returning to perform patient contact.)
- Perform hand hygiene after contact with blood, body fluids, mucous membranes, nonintact skin, secretions, excretions, or wound dressings; after contact with inanimate surfaces or articles in a patient room; and immediately after gloves are removed.
- When hands are visibly soiled or contaminated with blood or body fluids, wash them with either a nonantimicrobial or an antimicrobial soap and water.
- When hands are not visibly soiled or contaminated with blood or body fluids, use an alcohol-based, waterless antiseptic agent to perform hand hygiene (WHO, 2009).
- Wash hands with nonantimicrobial soap and water if contact with spores (e.g., C. diff) is likely to have occurred.
- Do not wear artificial fingernails or extenders if duties include direct contact with patients at high risk for infection and associated adverse outcomes.
- Wear gloves when touching blood, body fluids, secretions, excretions, nonintact skin, mucous membranes, or contaminated items or surfaces is likely. Remove gloves and perform hand

hygiene between patient care encounters and when going from a contaminated to a clean body site.

- Wear personal protective equipment (PPE) when the anticipated patient interaction indicates that contact with blood or body fluids may occur.
- A private room is unnecessary unless the patient's hygiene is unacceptable (e.g., uncontained secretions, excretions, or wound drainage).
- Discard all contaminated sharp instruments and needles in a puncture-resistant container. Health care facilities must make available needleless devices. Any needles should be disposed of uncapped, or a mechanical safety device is activated for covering the needle.
- Respiratory hygiene/cough etiquette: Have patients cover the nose/mouth when coughing or sneezing; use tissues to contain respiratory secretions and dispose in nearest waste container; perform hand hygiene after contacting respiratory secretions and contaminated objects/materials; contain respiratory secretions with procedure or surgical mask; spatial separation of at least 3 feet away from others if coughing.

Transmission-Based Precautions (Tier Two) for Use with Specific Types of Patients

Category	Infection/Condition	Barrier Protection
Airborne precautions (droplet nuclei smaller than 5 microns)	Measles, chickenpox (varicella), disseminated varicella zoster, pulmonary or laryngeal tuberculosis	Private room, negative-pressure airflow of at least 6-12 exchanges per hour via high-efficiency particulate air (HEPA) filtration; mask or respiratory protection device; N95 respirator (depending on condition)
Droplet precautions (droplets larger than 5 microns; being within 3 feet of the patient)	Diphtheria (pharyngeal), rubella, streptococcal pharyngitis, pneumonia or scarlet fever in infants and young children, pertussis, mumps, mycoplasma pneumonia, meningococcal pneumonia or sepsis, pneumonic plague	Private room or cohort patients; mask or respirator required (depending on condition) (refer to agency policy)

Continued

	Transmission-Based Precautions (Tier Two) for Use with Specific Types of Patients—Cont'd	
Category	Infection/Condition	Barrier Protection
Contact precautions (direct patient or environmental contact)	Colonization or infection with multidrug-resistant organisms, such as VRE and MRSA, *Clostridium difficile*, shigella, and other enteric pathogens; major wound infections; herpes simplex; scabies; varicella zoster (disseminated); respiratory syncytial virus in infants, young children, or immunocompromised adults	Private room or cohort patients (see agency policy); gloves; gowns (patients may leave their room for procedures or therapy if infectious material is contained or covered, placed in a clean gown, and if hands are cleaned)
Protective environment	Allogeneic hematopoietic stem cell transplants	Private room; positive airflow with 12 or more air exchanges per hour; HEPA filtration for incoming air; mask to be worn by patient when out of room

MRSA, Methicillin-resistant *Staphylococcus aureus*; *VRE*, vancomycin-resistant enterococcus.

Adapted from Centers for Disease Control and Prevention, Hospital Infection Control Practice Advisory Committee: Guidelines for isolation precautions in hospitals, *MMWR Morb Mortal Wkly Rep* 57/RR-16:39, 2007.

Special Precautions: Written by the Centers for Disease Control and Prevention (CDC) for certain diseases such as Ebola. See the CDC website (www.cdc.gov/infectioncontrol) for specifics on these special types of isolation.

PROTECTIVE ISOLATION

- Used for patients with compromised immune system.
- Protects the patient from microorganisms in the environment.
- Diligent handwashing is essential before patient care.
- Private room is necessary.
- A positive pressure room with a high-efficiency particulate air filtration system may be required.
- Precautions may include:
  - Masks for anyone entering the room, or for the patient when leaving the room
  - No live plants, fresh flowers, fresh raw fruit or vegetables, sushi, or blue cheese may be brought into the room, because these items may expose the patient to bacteria or fungi.

MEDICAL ASEPSIS VERSUS SURGICAL ASEPSIS

Medical Asepsis	Surgical Asepsis
• Perform diligent hand hygiene to assist in interrupting the chain of infection. • Avoid allowing soiled items such as linen to touch clothing to decrease the chance of spreading infectious material to other patients.	• Perform hand hygiene before sterile procedures. • Ensure that sterile objects touch only other sterile objects to maintain a sterile environment. • Open a sterile package away from the body to avoid contamination.

Continued

MEDICAL ASEPSIS VERSUS SURGICAL ASEPSIS—Cont'd

Medical Asepsis	Surgical Asepsis
• Keep soiled items off the floor to decrease the chance of contamination.	• Keep sterile surfaces dry. Avoid spilling liquids on a cloth or paper that is used as a sterile field. Fluids give organisms a means of transportation.
• Teach patients the proper use of tissues to cover sneezes and coughs. Prevent patients from coughing, sneezing, or breathing directly on others.	• Keep all sterile items above the waistline to ensure the sterile object is kept in sight.
• Avoid shaking linens to decrease the chance of infectious particles becoming airborne.	• Avoid coughing, talking, sneezing, or reaching across the sterile field.
• Clean from less soiled to more soiled areas to avoid increasing contamination.	• Face the sterile field. Never turn your back on or walk away from a sterile field.
• Place items that are moist from body fluids in the appropriate receptacle immediately. Wrap heavily soiled items in plastic to prevent direct contact with the substance by others.	• Keep items sterile that are used to enter a normally sterile environment (e.g., those that penetrate the skin or body). This includes dressings, needles, and catheter tubes.
• Pour liquids (e.g., bath water, mouthwash) directly into the drain to avoid splashing.	• Use dry, sterile forceps when necessary.

MEDICAL ASEPSIS VERSUS SURGICAL ASEPSIS—Cont'd

Medical Asepsis	Surgical Asepsis
• Sterilize items suspected of being contaminated. • Maintain personal hygiene. Keep fingernails short, keep hair short or pulled back, and avoid wearing rings with grooves or stones, which can harbor microorganisms. • Follow agency guidelines for standard and transmission-based precautions carefully.	• Remember that the outer 1 inch edge of a sterile field is contaminated. • Consider an object contaminated rather than sterile if there is any doubt.

From Yoost BL, Crawford LR: *Fundamentals of nursing: active learning for collaborative practice,* ed 2, St. Louis, 2020, Elsevier.

For additional information on infection control, consult the following:

Centers for Disease Control and Prevention (CDC). www.cdc.gov.

Phillips N: *Berry & Kohn's operating room technique,* ed 13, St. Louis, 2017, Elsevier.

Perry AG, Potter PA, Ostendorf WR: *Clinical nursing skills and techniques,* ed 9, St. Louis, 2018, Elsevier.

Potter PA, Perry AG, Stockert PA, Hall AM: *Fundamentals of nursing,* ed 10, St. Louis, 2021, Elsevier.

Rothrock JC, McEwen DR: *Alexander's care of the patient in surgery,* ed 16, St. Louis, 2019, Elsevier.

World Health Organization (WHO): *WHO guidelines on hand hygiene in healthcare,* Geneva, Switzerland. 2009, WHO Press.

Yoost BL, Crawford LR: *Fundamentals of nursing: active learning for collaborative practice,* ed 2, St. Louis, 2020, Elsevier.

CHAPTER 22

Mobility and Positioning

TYPES OF JOINTS
Primary Joint Classifications

Functional Name	Structural Name	Degree of Movement Permitted	Example
Synarthroses	Fibrous	Immovable	Sutures of the skull
Amphiarthroses	Cartilaginous	Slightly movable	Pubic symphysis
Diarthroses	Synovial	Freely movable	Shoulder joint

From Patton KT, Thibodeau GA: *Anatomy and physiology,* ed 9, St. Louis, 2016, Mosby.

Types of Synovial Joints

Types	Examples	Structure	Movement
Uniaxial			Around one axis; in one place
Hinge	Elbow joint	Spool-shaped process fits into a concave socket	Flexion and extension only
Pivot	Joint between the first and second cervical vertebrae	Arch-shaped process fits around a peglike process	Rotation
Biaxial			Around two axes, perpendicular to each other; in two planes
Saddle	Thumb joint between the first metacarpal and carpal bone	Saddle-shaped bone fits into a socket that is concave-convex-concave	Flexion, extension in one plane; abduction, adduction in the other plane; opposing the thumb to the fingers

Continued

Types of Synovial Joints—Cont'd

Types	Examples	Structure	Movement
Condyloid (ellipsoidal)	Joint between the radius and carpal bones	Oval condyle fits into an elliptical socket	Flexion, extension in one plane; abduction, adduction in the other plane
Multiaxial			Around many axes
Ball and socket	Shoulder joint and hip	Ball-shaped process fits into a concave socket	Widest range of movement: flexion, extension, abduction, adduction, rotation, circumduction
Gliding	Joints between the articular facets of adjacent vertebrae; joints between the carpal and tarsal bones	Relatively flat articulating surfaces	Gliding movements without any angular or circular movements

Adapted from Patton KT, Thibodeau GA: *Anatomy and physiology*, ed 9, St. Louis, 2016, Mosby.

POSITIONING

Supine: Patient lies flat on back

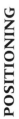

Prone: Patient lies face-down

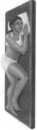

Semi-Fowler: Patient semisitting with head elevated

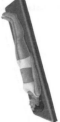

Fowler: Patient in sitting position with pillow supporting thigh and legs

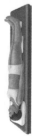

Sim's: Patient in semiprone position lying on the left side

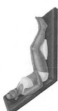

Side-lying: Patient lying on side

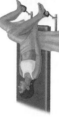

Dorsal recumbent: Patient lying supine with legs bent

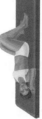

Lithotomy: Patient lying supine with feet in stirrups

Knee-chest: Patient lying in prone position with buttocks and knees drawn to the chest

Trendelenburg's: Patient lying supine with legs elevated higher than head

(From Yoost BL, Crawford LR: *Fundamentals of nursing: active learning for collaborative practice,* ed 2, St. Louis, 2020, Elsevier.)

TRANSFERS
Mechanical Lifts

- **Mobile hydraulic lifts:** also known as Hoyer lifts or powered full-body lifts. The patient is rolled onto a full-body sling and lifted. Can be used to lift patient off the bed for linen changes, to transfer a patient to a different bed or stretcher, or to transfer the patient from bed to chair or toilet. Can also be used with an ambulation sling for patients who are unsteady.

- **Ceiling lifts:** ceiling-mounted track with a sling. Similar to the mobile hydraulic lift, but patient can only be moved within the room that has the track. May be used with an ambulation sling.

- **Stand-up assist lifts:** hydraulic sling lift for partial-weight-bearing and cooperative patients. The patient stands on the lift and is secured with a harness for transfers.

- **Transfer chairs:** convertible chair-stretcher devices for non–weight-bearing or immobile patients. The patient can be placed in a lying or sitting position without moving to another surface.

- **Lateral assist lifts:** motorized or hand-cranked transfer devices built onto a stretcher. They are designed for immobile patients who are unable to assist in transfers. They allow the space between the bed and the stretcher to be bridged without the caregiver reaching or pulling, avoiding potential injuries.

Transfer Assistive Devices

- Special mattresses or beds designed to minimize transfer and repositioning. Several types are available:
  - Surface redesign mattress has rotating surfaces that eliminate the need to move the patient (bed

surface moves instead) and has an air cushion that eliminates friction during movement.

- A Gatch bed has a frame that is made in three sections, which permits raising the head, foot, and middle of the bed.
- A specialized foam mattress reduces pressure to avoid or alleviate pressure injuries.
- A foam or gel combination mattress reduces pressure on bony prominences.
- A low-air-loss bed uses multiple air-filled cushions and various amounts of air, can support a wide range of patient weights, and reduces pressure to avoid or alleviate pressure injuries.
- An air-fluidized bed uses airflow to move silicone particles in the bed, creating a watery, fluidlike movement and resulting in lower pressure to avoid or alleviate pressure injuries.

- Trapeze Bar
  - Fastens to an overhead bar that is attached to the bed frame.
  - Used for patients with upper extremity strength.
  - Patients can use a trapeze bar to assist with repositioning.
  - Use of the bar decreases the risk of shearing.
  - Musculoskeletal strength increases, because the bar accommodates upper extremity exercises.
  - Having a trapeze bar available to the patient promotes independence.
- Transfer or slide board
  - A transfer or slide board is made of plasticlike material that reduces friction.
  - Linens easily slide over the board, facilitating bed linen changes.
  - Patient can slide from bed to chair or bed to stretcher.

- Patients can be repositioned or transferred with a minimum of force required.
- Friction-reducing sheet
  - Similar to transfer or slide boards:
    - Made of a specialized material that reduces shear and friction.
    - When placed under a patient, the sheet minimizes the force required for repositioning or transfer.
    - Prevents friction injuries to the patient.

Safe Patient Handling and Mobility Algorithms

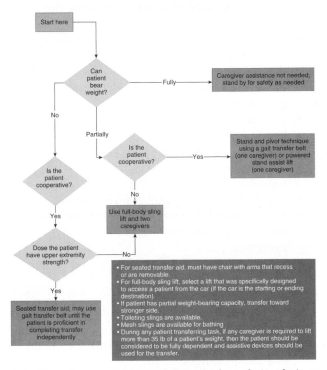

Algorithm 1: Transfer to and from bed to chair, chair to toilet, chair to chair, or car to chair. (Courtesy U.S. Department of Veterans Affairs.)

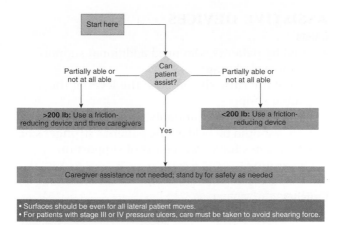

Algorithm 2: Lateral transfer to and from bed to stretcher or trolley. (Courtesy U.S. Department of Veterans Affairs.)

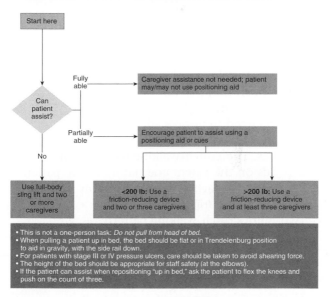

Algorithm 3: Reposition in bed side to side, up in bed. (Courtesy U.S. Department of Veterans Affairs.)

ASSISTIVE DEVICES

Canes

- Used by patients who need additional support when ambulating.
- Top of the cane should be at the level of the patient's hip.
- Arm should be comfortably bent.
- Canes should be held on the patient's stronger side.
- Quad canes have four points of support on the ground.

Crutches

- Underarm crutches should be fitted to allow approximately 2 inches or 3 finger widths of space between the top of the crutch and the axilla when the crutch is placed slightly in front of and 6 inches to the side of the foot. The patient's elbow should be comfortably bent.
- Forearm or Lofstrand crutches are used for patients with long-term or permanent impairment. Forearm crutches are designed with a handgrip and a metal cuff that partially or completely surrounds the lower arm.
- Patients need to possess adequate upper body strength and coordination when using all types of crutches. The crutch-walking pattern employed depends on the extent and nature of the patient's disability. For each pattern the patient starts with crutches in the tripod position.
- Two-point crutch-walking pattern:
  - Used by patients who can bear partial weight on either or both lower extremities.
  - Provides stability and support for ambulation.
  - Patients move one crutch forward simultaneously with the opposite leg.
  - Provides a wide base of support.

- Three-point crutch walking:
  - Used by patients who have injury to one leg.
  - Both crutches are placed forward, and patients swing their legs to the center of the crutches, bearing weight on only the uninjured leg.
  - A similar crutch-walking pattern is referred to as a swing-to gait used by paraplegics. Crutches are placed forward and the patient swings both legs to the center of the crutches.
- Four-point crutch gait:
  - Requires partial weight bearing on both lower extremities.
  - Provides more stability than the two-point pattern, because only one of four points of support is lifted off the floor at any time.
  - The patient moves one crutch forward, followed by the opposing leg, and repeats the pattern by moving the opposite crutch and then the leg forward.

Walkers

- Come with and without wheels.
- Provide more support than a cane.
- Can be used for patients who have weakness or balance problems or who are recovering from back or leg injuries.
- Should be waist high and slightly wider than the patient.
- A walker without wheels is used in a manner similar to crutches. This type of device can be used in the same manner as a three-point crutch gait. The patient lifts the walker forward one step and then swings or steps both legs into it.
- A wheeled walker is pushed along as the patient walks within the walker frame. Patient using a wheeled walker must have good balance.

For additional information on mobility and positioning,
consult the following:

National Institute for Occupational Safety and Health (NIOSH): Safe patient
   handling and mobility, 2017. www.cdc.gov/niosh/topics/safepatient/
   default.html.
Patton KT, Thibodeau GA: *Anatomy and physiology,* ed 9, St. Louis, 2016,
   Elsevier.
Perry AG, Potter PA, Ostendorf WR: *Clinical nursing skills and techniques,* ed 9,
   St. Louis, 2018, Elsevier.
Potter PA, Perry AG, Stockert PA, Hall AM: *Fundamentals of nursing,* ed 10,
   St. Louis, 2021, Elsevier.
Yoost BL, Crawford LR: *Fundamentals of nursing: active learning for collab-
   orative practice,* ed 2, St. Louis, 2020, Elsevier.

CHAPTER 23

Personal Care

BATHING AND HYGIENE

Assessment of Hygiene Needs

- Assess self-care abilities during the initial patient interview.
- Assessment of the patient's current hygiene needs is performed with each encounter.
- If the patient is unable to care for hygiene needs, assess whether a complete bed bath, a partial bed bath, a sink bath, or a shower is indicated. Incorporate oral, eye, ear, nose, hand, foot, and perineal care, as well as shaving and massage, into the hygiene plan.
- Cleansing of the skin is an important component of patient care. Bathing rids the skin of bacteria, odor, and dead skin.

Bathing Basics

- After initial assessment by the RN, bathing may be delegated to the unlicensed assistive personnel (UAP).
- Offer a urinal or bedpan before beginning a bed bath.
- Prepare all items needed ahead of time.

- Test the water temperature to make sure it is not too hot, from 40.5°C–43.3°C (105°F–110°F), but warm enough for the patient to bathe comfortably.
- Allow the patient to participate as much as possible.
- A complete bed bath provides the opportunity for a thorough skin assessment.
- Talk to the patient throughout the bath, explaining the procedure and asking assessment questions.
- Change the water when it becomes soiled or cools off.
- Work from the cleanest parts of the body to the dirtiest, starting with the eyes and working downward to the feet and buttocks.
- Dry each area after washing and rinsing, making sure to thoroughly dry skin folds under arms, breasts, abdomen, and groin, and between the buttocks and toes.
- Provide passive range of motion if the patient is unable to perform active range of motion.
- Apply lotion to dry areas unless contraindicated.
- Provide patient with a clean gown after the bath.
- Make the bed with fresh linens after the bath and whenever the linens become soiled.

Bathing
- A complete bed bath is performed for patients who are bedridden or are not able to care for themselves.
- A partial bed bath may be necessary when a patient has been incontinent, or when a patient wants to wash before breakfast. Any portion of the complete bed bath may be given, depending on the patient circumstances.
- Patients with extremely dry skin may not require a complete bath every day. Only soiled areas are washed in between complete baths.
- Patients who are allowed out of bed may prefer to wash while standing at the sink or sitting in a chair

with a bath basin on the bedside table in front
of them.
- Some hospital units have shower rooms.
Assessment is necessary to determine whether the
patient is strong enough to stand in the shower. An
order from the PCP for a shower may be necessary.
- In long-term care, shower chairs are utilized so that
patients can sit and be washed in the shower by a
caregiver.

Perineal Care
- Perineal care cleanses the genitals, urinary meatus,
and anus. It may be delegated to the UAP after
assessment by the nurse.
- Some patients prefer a caregiver of the same gender
for personal or religious reasons.
- Patients who are dependent for their hygienic
needs, who are incontinent, or who have a urinary
catheter need special attention to their
perineal care.
- Perineal care is provided during a complete bed
bath but may be necessary more often.
- Always wear gloves when providing perineal care.
- The male is washed with circular motions starting
at the urinary meatus, then with long firm strokes
down the shaft of the penis. If the male is
uncircumcised, gently retract the foreskin before
washing, Reposition the foreskin after drying
the penis.
- The female is washed from the front toward the
back of the perineum using downward strokes.
A clean portion of the washcloth is used with each
stroke.

Hand and Foot Care
- Hands and feet can be washed as part of a complete
bath or can be done separately as needed.

- If a patient has diabetes or peripheral vascular disease, do not soak the hands and feet as this may cause dryness, skin breakdown, or infection.
- Do not cut the toenails of a patient with diabetes or peripheral vascular disease. A referral to a diabetic foot care specialist may be necessary.
- If not contraindicated, hand and foot care may be delegated to the UAP.
- Soak the hand or foot in warm water for 10 minutes. Wash, rinse, and dry the hand or foot.
- Trim the nails straight across if not contraindicated. Then use an emery board to smooth the edges.
- Apply lotion if desired.

Massage
- Massage can be performed as part of a bed bath or at any time during patient care to provide relaxation, complimentary pain relief, increased circulation, and to promote sleep.
- Techniques:
  - Effleurage: firm, long, continuous stokes along the length of the back.
  - Petrissage: kneading motion along the back and shoulders with the fingers and thumb.
  - Tapotement: tapping with the palm or ulnar side of the hand to stimulate the skin. Should not be performed over the kidney area.

Hair Care
- Hair care may be delegated to the UAP.
- A patient's hair should be combed or brushed at least daily.
- If a patient's hair is dirty, oily, or matted with blood, a shampoo might be necessary.
- Remove hearing aids before shampooing a patient's hair.

- Shampooing can be accomplished by several methods:
  - If the patient is strong enough to shower, shampooing can occur during the shower.
  - Some facilities have shampoo basins so bedridden patients can have their hair washed.
  - Shampoo caps are available in some facilities. Hair is lathered under the cap then toweled dry and combed.
  - Dry or no-rinse shampoo may be used to decrease oil in patients who cannot have their hair washed.
- Towel dry and comb the patient's hair after shampooing.

Oral Care
- Oral care for all patients (natural teeth and dentures) may be delegated to the UAP and should be done at least twice daily.
- Patients on anticoagulant therapy should use a soft bristle brush.
- Brushing the teeth, gums, and tongue, as well as rinsing with mouthwash, are components of oral care.
- An oral sponge called a toothette can be used for patients who need frequent oral care or who are unconscious.
- During oral care, keep suction equipment at the bedside of all patients who have a diminished gag reflex or who are unconscious.

Eye Care
- Wash the patient's eyes using a clean washcloth and warm water (no soap) starting at the inner canthus and wiping outward. Use a clean part of the cloth for each eye.

- If the patient wears eyeglasses, they can be cleansed with liquid soap and water and dried with a soft cloth.
- If the patient wears contact lenses that are inserted and removed daily:
  - Store the lenses in manufacturer recommended solution in a contact lens case labeled with the patient's name when not in use.
  - Wash hands before handling the lenses.
  - Always insert and remove the same lens first (for example, always start with the right lens). This helps avoid confusion and accidently inserting the wrong lens into an eye.
  - Some right eye lenses have a small mark to avoid inserting the wrong lens.
  - If the patient is able to insert and remove the lenses, allow their use during hospitalization.
  - If a patient is unable to care for contact lenses, encourage them to switch to glasses during hospitalization.
  - Discard the lens solution and clean the case after insertion.
  - Upon removal of lenses, store them in fresh solution in the clean lens container.
- For emergency removal of contact lenses:
  - Soft lenses: With gloves on, pull down the lower eyelid with your nondominant hand while the patient looks up. Use the thumb and forefinger of your dominant hand to pinch the edges of the contact together for removal.
  - Hard lenses: With gloves on using your dominant hand, place the thumb below the patient's lower eyelid and the index finger on the upper lid. Separate the lids and have the patient blink. The lens should pop out.

Nose Care
- Patients who are unable to blow their nose may need moist secretions removed by suction.
- Dried secretions can be removed with a moistened cotton tip applicator. Never insert the applicator into the nares further than the depth of the cotton tip.
- Oxygen dries nasal passages, especially at higher levels. Humidification may help alleviate this problem.
- Patients with tubes in their nose (nasogastric feeding tubes or suction tubes) may have crusting around the tube. This can be removed with saline-moistened gauze or cotton-tipped applicators.

Ear Care
- Ears are washed with soap and water and dried with a towel during the bath.
- Patients with cerumen buildup may have special drops ordered that soften the wax before irrigation is performed. Do not try to remove the wax with a cotton-tip applicator.
- Hearing aids:
  - If a patient wears hearing aids, they should be worn while in the hospital so that the patient can hear what is being said.
  - Keep hearing aids dry. Remove them before bathing or shampooing a patient. Clean with a dry cloth.
  - Help the patient change hearing aid batteries as necessary.
  - Hearing aids are costly and should be stored in a container with the patient's name when not in use.

Shaving
- Assess the patient's personal preferences before shaving.

- Shaving may be delegated to the UAP after assessment.
- Some men have facial hair that they do not wish to shave. Never shave a patient's beard or mustache without the patient's or family's permission.
- Many men shave their faces daily.
- Many women shave their legs and axilla. Some women have facial hair that they prefer to shave.
- Electric razors should be used for any patient on anticoagulant therapy. Hospitals usually have inexpensive electric razors for patient use. Razors should never be shared.
- Bladed safety razors may be used when not contraindicated.
- Dispose of used safety razors in the sharps container.

ELIMINATION
Toileting
- Provide for patient privacy during toileting.
- Patients on bed rest or those who are incontinent should be on a toileting schedule. The patient is offered a urinal or placed on the bedpan, bedside commode, or toilet at specified intervals.
- Toileting may be delegated to the UAP after initial assessment of the patient's status.
- Always wear gloves when assisting patients with elimination.

Intake and Output
- Documentation of intake and output (I&O) is included in most patient EHRs.
- Fluid intake is recorded in mL and includes oral fluid, tube feedings, and IV fluids.
- Output is measured in mL and includes urine, drainage from wounds, emesis, liquid feces, nasogastric suction secretions, and blood.

- Some patients are on fluid restrictions, and it is imperative that their I&O are documented accurately.

AVERAGE DAILY FLUID INTAKE AND OUTPUT

Intake (mL)		Output (mL)	
Fluids	1600	Urine	1500
Food	700	Feces	200
Metabolism	200	Skin, including perspiration	500
		Lungs	300
Total intake	2500	Total output	2500

From Yoost BL, Crawford LR: *Fundamentals of nursing: active learning for collaborative practice,* ed 2, St. Louis, 2020, Elsevier.

Bedpan, Urinal, Urine Hat, Bedside Commode

- Patients who are on bed rest may need to use a bedpan or urinal for elimination.
- Fracture bedpans are smaller and may be used for patients who are unable to be raised high enough to sit on a regular bedpan.
- Urinals are used for male patients who are unable to get out of bed to use the bathroom. The penis is placed in the opening of the urinal and the patient urinates. The urinal is shaped so that the urine flows into the container without spilling.
- A urine hat is a measuring device that is placed on a toilet or bedside commode. It has graduated markings so that urine or liquid stool can be measured. Bedpans, fracture bedpans, and urinals also have markings so that urine and stool can be measured.

- Bedside commodes are chairs with a toilet seat top and a container underneath for collection of urine and stool. They are used for patients who are allowed up in a chair but are unable to walk to the bathroom.

Urinary catheters
- Basic care
  - Perform hand hygiene before catheter insertion or care.
  - Always wear gloves when providing catheter care.
  - Avoid raising the drainage bag above the level of the bladder.
  - Empty the drainage bag at least every 8 hours.
- Condom
  - A new condom catheter is placed over the penis daily.
  - Perform perineal care before placing the new catheter.
  - Assess the skin during perineal care.
  - Apply skin barrier to the penis and allow it to dry.
  - Catheter is attached to a drainage bag.
- Indwelling
  - Provide perineal care before inserting the catheter.
  - Sterile aseptic technique is used when inserting the catheter.
  - Double lumen catheter is used to drain urine over a period of time or to provide an accurate measurement of urinary output. The second lumen is used to fill a balloon in the bladder to hold the catheter in.
  - Triple lumen catheters are used when bladder irrigation is necessary.

- Indwelling catheters are attached to a drainage bag.
- When a patient has an indwelling catheter, perineal care should be performed at least daily. After perineal care, hold the catheter near the urinary meatus and wash the catheter with a clean cloth and soap and water from the meatus away from the body at least 4 inches. Rinse and dry.
- Straight
  - Provide perineal care before inserting the catheter.
  - Sterile aseptic technique is used when inserting the catheter.
  - One-time or short-term catheter is used to obtain a sterile urine sample, assess residual urine after voiding, or relieve bladder distension.
- Suprapubic
  - Catheter is placed surgically through the abdominal wall into the bladder in patients with urethral obstructions.
  - The catheter may be secured using tape, sutures, or a balloon inside the bladder.
  - For established catheters, cleanse around the site in a circular motion daily with soap and water, starting at the catheter and working outward. Use a clean cloth to wash the catheter, starting at the insertion site and working away from the body.
  - Catheter is attached to a drainage bag.

ALTERED BOWEL ELIMINATION PATTERNS

- Constipation
  - Infrequent or difficult bowel movements. Less than 3 bowel movements per week.

- Causes: Reabsorption of too much water in the lower bowel as a result of medication such as narcotics, ignoring the urge to defecate, immobility, chronic laxative abuse, low fluid intake, low fiber intake, aging, postoperative conditions, or pregnancy.
- Interventions: Increase fluids, fiber cereals, fruits and vegetables, and exercise, and avoid cheese.
- Impaction
  - Hard fecal mass in the rectum or colon; may have liquid stool passing around impaction.
  - Causes: Poor bowel habits, prolonged constipation, immobility, inadequate food or fluids, or barium in rectum.
  - Interventions: Digitally remove impaction, increase fluids and fiber, increase exercise, and institute bowel program.
- Diarrhea
  - Abnormal frequency or fluidity of stools.
  - Causes: Infection, anxiety, stress, medications, too many laxatives, or food or drug allergies or reactions.
  - Interventions: Add bulk or fiber to diet, maintain fluids and electrolytes, eat smaller bland meals. Avoid milk products, spices, gas-producing foods, and caffeine.
- Incontinence
  - Loss of voluntary control of feces.
  - Causes: Surgery, cancer, radiation treatment of rectum, paralysis, or aging.
  - Interventions: Bowel training, regular mealtimes, regular elimination times.
- Obstruction
  - Occurs when the lumen of the bowel narrows or closes completely
  - Causes: External compression can be caused by tumor; internal narrowing can be caused by impacted feces.

- Interventions: Remove impaction or tumor.
- Paralytic ileus
  - Occurs when the bowel has decreased motility and peristalsis stops.
  - Causes: Surgery, long-term narcotic use, or complete obstruction
  - Interventions: Specific action depends on the cause of the ileus.

For additional information on personal care, consult the following:

Ignatavicius DD, Workman ML, Rebar CR, et al: *Medical-surgical nursing: patient-centered collaborative care,* ed 9, St. Louis, 2018, Elsevier.

Lewis SL, Bucher L, Heitkemper MM, et al: *Medical-surgical nursing,* ed 10, St. Louis, 2017, Elsevier.

Perry AG, Potter PA, Ostendorf WR: *Clinical nursing skills and techniques,* ed 9, St. Louis, 2018, Elsevier.

Potter PA, Perry AG, Stockert PA, Hall AM: *Fundamentals of nursing,* ed 10, St. Louis, 2021, Elsevier.

Yoost BL, Crawford LR: *Fundamentals of nursing: active learning for collaborative practice,* ed 2, St. Louis, 2020, Elsevier.

CHAPTER 24

Wound Care

FOCUSED WOUND ASSESSMENT QUESTIONS

- How long has this wound been present?
- What do you think caused this wound?
- Have you ever had a wound like this before?
- What are you doing for this wound at home? What are you using to clean the wound? What have you put on it?
- Have you noticed any changes in the appearance of the wound or the skin around it?
- How much wound drainage is there? Has the amount, color, or odor of the drainage changed? How often do you need to change the bandage at home?
- Do you live alone? Do you have anyone who helps you at home?
- Is the cost of caring for this wound difficult for you to manage?

PRESSURE INJURY RISK ASSESSMENT
Standardized Risk Assessment Scales

- Standardized scales are used to predict pressure injury risk in hospitalized patients.

- Two common scales are the Braden scale for predicting pressure sore risk and the Norton pressure ulcer scale.

BRADEN SCALE FOR PREDICTING PRESSURE SORE RISK					
Patient's name		Evaluator's name		Date of assessment	
SENSORY PERCEPTION Ability to respond meaningfully to pressure-related discomfort	**1. Completely Limited** Unresponsive (does not moan, flinch, or gasp) to painful stimuli. Cannot communicate discomfort except by moaning or restlessness. OR Limited ability to feel pain over most of body.	**2. Very Limited** Responds only to painful stimuli. Cannot communicate discomfort except by moaning or restlessness. OR Has a sensory impairment that limits the ability to feel pain or discomfort over ½ of body.	**3. Slightly Limited** Responds to verbal commands, but cannot always communicate discomfort or the need to be turned. OR Has some sensory impairment that limits ability to feel pain or discomfort in 1 or 2 extremities.	**4. No Impairment** Responds to verbal commands. Has no sensory deficit that would limit ability to feel or voice pain and discomfort.	
MOISTURE Degree to which skin is exposed to moisture	**1. Constantly Moist** Skin is kept moist almost constantly by perspiration, urine, etc. Dampness is detected every time patient is moved or turned.	**2. Very Moist** Skin is often, but not always moist. Linen must be changed at least once a shift.	**3. Occasionally Moist** Skin is occasionally moist, requiring an extra linen change approximately once a day.	**4. Rarely Moist** Skin is usually dry; linen only requires changing at routine intervals.	
ACTIVITY Degree of physical activity	**1. Bedfast** Confined to bed.	**2. Chairfast** Ability to walk severely limited or non-existent. Cannot bear own weight and/or must be assisted into chair or wheelchair.	**3. Walks Occasionally** Walks occasionally during day, but for very short distances, with or without assistance. Spends majority of each shift in bed or chair.	**4. Walks Frequently** Walks outside room at least twice a day and inside room at least once every 2 hours during waking hours.	
MOBILITY Ability to change and control body position	**1. Completely Immobile** Does not make even slight changes in body or extremity position without assistance.	**2. Very Limited** Makes occasional slight changes in body or extremity position, but unable to make frequent or significant changes independently.	**3. Slightly Limited** Makes frequent though slight changes in body or extremity position independently.	**4. No Limitation** Makes major and frequent changes in position without assistance.	
NUTRITION Usual food intake pattern	**1. Very Poor** Never eats a complete meal. Rarely eats more than ⅓ of food offered. Eats 2 servings or less of protein (meat or dairy products) per day. Takes fluids poorly. Does not take a liquid dietary supplement. OR Is NPO and/or maintained on clear liquids or IVs for more than 5 days.	**2. Probably Inadequate** Rarely eats a complete meal and generally eats only about ½ of any food offered. Protein intake includes only 3 servings of meat or dairy products per day. Occasionally will take a dietary supplement. OR Receives less than optimum amount of liquid diet or tube feeding.	**3. Adequate** Eats over half of most meals. Eats a total of 4 servings of protein (meat, dairy products) per day. Occasionally will refuse a meal, but will usually take a supplement when offered. OR Is on a tube feeding or TPN regimen that probably meets most of nutritional needs.	**4. Excellent** Eats most of every meal. Never refuses a meal. Usually eats a total of 4 or more servings of meat and dairy products. Occasionally eats between meals. Does not require supplementation.	
FRICTION and SHEAR	**1. Problem** Requires moderate to maximum assistance in moving. Complete lifting without sliding against sheets is impossible. Frequently slides down in bed or chair, requiring frequent repositioning with maximum assistance. Spasticity, contractures, or agitation leads to almost constant friction.	**2. Potential Problem** Moves feebly or requires minimum assistance. During a move, skin probably slides to some extent against sheets, chair restraints, or other devices. Maintains relatively good position in chair or bed most of the time but occasionally slides down.	**3. No Apparent Problem** Moves in bed and in chair independently and has sufficient muscle strength to lift up completely during move. Maintains good position in bed or chair.		
				Total score	

The Braden scale for predicting pressure sore risk. A score lower than 18 places the patient at risk for pressure injury. (Copyright, Barbara Braden and Nancy Bergstrom, 1988. Reprinted with permission. All rights reserved.)

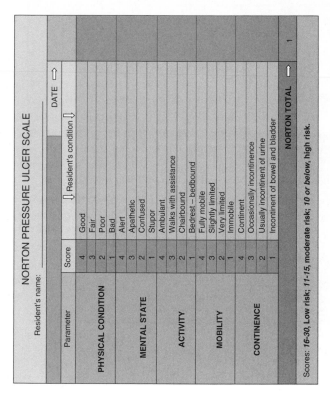

NORTON PRESSURE ULCER SCALE		
Resident's name:		
		DATE ⇧
Parameter	Score	⇩ Resident's condition ⇩
PHYSICAL CONDITION	4	Good
	3	Fair
	2	Poor
	1	Bad
MENTAL STATE	4	Alert
	3	Apathetic
	2	Confused
	1	Stupor
ACTIVITY	4	Ambulant
	3	Walks with assistance
	2	Chairbound
	1	Bedrest – bedbound
MOBILITY	4	Fully mobile
	3	Slightly limited
	2	Very limited
	1	Immobile
CONTINENCE	4	Continent
	3	Occasionally incontinence
	2	Usually incontinent of urine
	1	Incontinent of bowel and bladder
		NORTON TOTAL ⇧ 1
Scores: *16-30, Low risk; 11-15, moderate risk; 10 or below, high risk.*		

Norton scale.

(Adapted from Norton D, McLaren R, Exton-Smith AN: *An investigation of geriatric nursing problems in hospital,* London, 1962, Churchill Livingstone.)

Possible Sites of Pressure Injuries

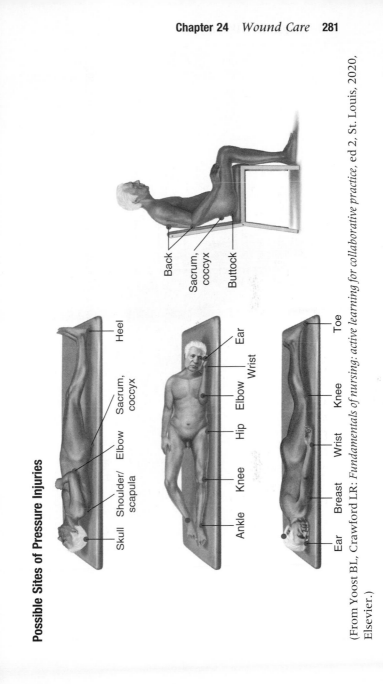

(From Yoost BL, Crawford LR: *Fundamentals of nursing: active learning for collaborative practice*, ed 2, St. Louis, 2020, Elsevier.)

Friction and Shear

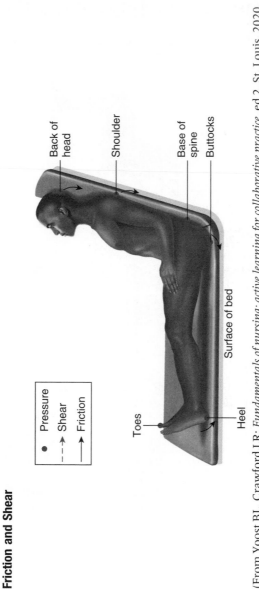

(From Yoost BL, Crawford LR: *Fundamentals of nursing: active learning for collaborative practice*, ed 2, St. Louis, 2020, Elsevier.)

CLASSIFICATION OF PRESSURE INJURIES

- Classified, or staged, according to the type of tissue visible in the wound bed.
- The National Pressure Ulcer Advisory Panel (NPUAP) updated the classifications in 2016.

Stage 1 Pressure Injury

- Nonblanchable erythema of intact skin characterized by intact, nonblistered skin with nonblanchable erythema, or persistent redness, in the area that has been exposed to pressure.

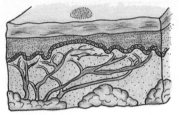

(From Potter PA, Perry AG, Stockert PA, Hall AM: Clinical companion for fundamentals of nursing: just the facts, ed 9, St. Louis, 2017, Elsevier; Perry AG, et al: *Clinical nursing skills and techniques*, ed 9, St. Louis, 2018, Elsevier.)

Stage 2 Pressure Injury

- Partial-thickness superficial skin loss with exposed dermis that involves the epidermis and/or dermis but does not extend below the level of the dermis.
- May also present as an intact or ruptured blister.

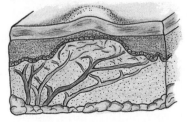

(From Potter PA, Perry AG, Stockert PA, Hall AM: Clinical companion for fundamentals of nursing: just the facts, ed 9, St. Louis, 2017, Elsevier; Perry AG, et al: *Clinical nursing skills and techniques*, ed 9, St. Louis, 2018, Elsevier.)

Stage 3 Pressure Injury

- Full-thickness wounds that extend into the subcutaneous tissue but do not extend through the fascia to muscle, bone, or connective tissue.
- May be undermining or tunneling present in the wound.

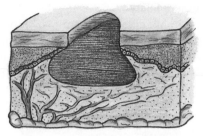

(From Potter PA, Perry AG, Stockert PA, Hall AM: Clinical companion for fundamentals of nursing: just the facts, ed 9, St. Louis, 2017, Elsevier; Perry AG, et al: *Clinical nursing skills and techniques*, ed 9, St. Louis, 2018, Elsevier.)

Stage 4 Pressure Injury

- Full-thickness skin and tissue loss that involves exposure of muscle, bone, or connective tissue, such as tendons or cartilage.

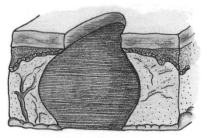

(From Potter PA, Perry AG, Stockert PA, Hall AM: Clinical companion for fundamentals of nursing: just the facts, ed 9, St. Louis, 2017, Elsevier; Perry AG, et al: *Clinical nursing skills and techniques*, ed 9, St. Louis, 2018, Elsevier.)

Unstageable Pressure Injury

- Full-thickness wound in which the amount of necrotic tissue, or eschar, in the wound bed makes it impossible to assess the depth of the wound or the involvement of underlying structures.

• The wound cannot be staged until the necrotic tissue is removed or debrided.

Deep Tissue Pressure Injury

• Persistent, nonblanchable discoloration is an area of intact skin that is purple or maroon or a blood-filled blister.

• The depth of tissue damage is not readily apparent on initial inspection; however, these injuries can progress rapidly, exposing deeper layers of tissue even if treated quickly and appropriately.

WOUND ASSESSMENT
Wound Assessment During a Dressing Change

• Location
  • Describe using clear anatomical terminology.
  • Mark the wound on an anatomical diagram.
• Size
  • Used to monitor wound healing.
  • Measured in centimeters and millimeters.
  • Always wear clean or sterile gloves, depending on the type of wound.
  • Width: measured laterally from left to right at the widest open part of the wound.
  • Length: measured top to bottom (or head to foot) at the longest open part of the wound.
  • Depth: measured by inserting a cotton-tipped applicator into the deepest part of the wound, marking the applicator level with the skin, then holding the applicator up to the tape measure to determine depth.
• Undermining
  • Measure the depth of the undermining by inserting a cotton-tipped applicator laterally at all locations where there is tissue loss under intact skin.
  • Describe the anatomical location of the undermining.

- Tunneling
  - Measure the depth of tunneling by inserting a cotton-tipped applicator into all locations where there is a narrow passage extending from the wound bed.
  - Describe the anatomical location of the tunneling.
- Drainage
  - Amount: small, moderate, large, or describe by size of discoloration on gauze.
  - Color: serous (clear), serosanguineous (pink to pale red), sanguineous (bright red), green, yellow.
  - Consistency: thick or thin, clots.
  - Odor: foul, no odor.
- Condition of wound edges and surrounding tissue
  - Maceration.
  - Signs of infection: redness, warmth.
- Wound bed
  - Granulation tissue: beefy red, shiny, moist.
  - Necrotic tissue: black or yellow.
  - Pale: lack of circulation.
  - Subcutaneous tissue visible.
  - Bone, muscle, or cartilage visible.
- Patient response
  - Note the patient's response to wound measurement and treatment.
  - If patient has severe pain during treatment, provide pharmacological and complimentary pain interventions before the next treatment.

Documentation
- Accurate documentation in the EHR includes:
  - Wound location, width, length, and depth, as well as any undermining or tunneling with locations and measurements.
  - The presence and characteristics of drainage.

- The condition of the wound bed and periwound area.
- Dressing changes or other treatments.
- The patient's response.

WOUND CARE
Types of Dressings
- Gauze
  - Many shapes and sizes.
  - Used to protect a wound and absorb drainage.
  - Disadvantages: not an effective barrier to infection, does not keep the wound bed moist, may be difficult to remove.
  - May be impregnated with antibiotics to prevent infection or petroleum to prevent the dressing from sticking to the wound.
  - May be used dry for absorption.
  - Wet to damp or dry dressing, use saline-moistened gauze, which is allowed to dry or partially dry. When removed, the dry dressing pulls necrotic tissue out of the wound.
- Transparent
  - Adhesive-backed polyurethane.
  - Prevents bacteria from entering the wound but allows oxygen and water vapor to move through the dressing.
  - Maintain a moist wound environment.
  - Cannot be used when there is more than a small amount of drainage.
  - Appropriate for autolytic debridement of a minimally draining wound that is not infected.
- Hydrocolloid
  - Occlusive, adhesive dressing that absorbs a small to moderate amount of drainage.
  - Changed every 5 to 7 days or when adhesive is loose.
  - Provide a moist wound environment.
  - Appropriate for autolytic debridement.

- Foam
  - Pull fluid away from the wound while maintaining a moist wound environment.
  - For wounds with moderate to heavy drainage.
  - Can be used over enzymatic debriding agents.
- Alginate
  - Used in wounds with heavy drainage.
  - Made from brown seaweed fibers and highly absorbant.
  - Nonadhesive, nonocclusive.
  - Can be combined with other types of dressings.
  - Helps stop bleeding.
- Gel
  - Adds moisture to wounds to create a moist environment.
  - Allows autolytic debridement and wound healing to occur.
  - Nonabsorbent therefore useful for wounds without exudate.

Wound Cleansing and Irrigation

- Most wounds are cleansed with sterile 0.9% normal saline solution.
- Some products such as povidone-iodine and hydrogen peroxide kill bacteria but are cytotoxic to healthy cells needed for wound healing.
- Wound irrigation is performed to clean a wound, apply heat, instill medication, remove debris and exudate, and remove bacteria.
- The solution is instilled with enough force to remove bacteria and exudate without damaging healthy tissue.
- Wound irrigation is a sterile procedure.
- Proper PPE (gown, gloves, goggles, mask) is necessary to protect the nurse from possible splashing of fluid.
- Irrigate from least contaminated area to most contaminated area.

- Use gauze to thoroughly dry the area around the wound with a patting motion. Redress the wound.

Other Wound Care Interventions

- Drains
  - Placed in surgical sites to drain blood, serum, and pus.
  - Color, consistency, and odor of drainage is assessed.
  - Jackson-Pratt (JP) drain: a closed-wound drainage system with a bulblike suction device that is emptied, measured, and compressed before replugging.
  - Hemovac drain: a closed-wound drainage system with a springlike suction device that is emptied, measured, and compressed before replugging.
  - Penrose drain: an open-wound drainage system with a flexible tube that drains excess fluid from a wound, usually abdominal. A sterile safety pin is placed through the drain to prevent the tube from slipping inside the wound. Drainage flows onto gauze bandages.
  - Cleanse around wound drainage tubing with a circular motion using sterile gauze and saline, starting near the tubing and working outward.
- Negative-pressure wound therapy
  - Wound vacuum-assisted closure device.
  - Removes exudate, stabilizes wound edges, and stimulates granulation tissue.
- Suture and staple care
  - Wounds may be closed with sutures, staples, Dermabond glue, or Steri-strips.
  - When there is an order for cleansing of an incision, start in the least contaminated area and work toward the most contaminated area,

usually starting near the incision line and working outward. Sterile gauze and saline are used.

- Cleanse the incision before and after staple or suture removal.
- Bandages and binders
  - Used to secure dressings, provide support and protection, apply pressure, and immobilize body parts.
  - Check five p's of circulation (pain, pallor, pulselessness, paresthesia, paralysis) within 30 minutes of applying bandages or binders.
  - Montgomery straps are sometimes used to hold abdominal dressings in place.
- Heat and cold therapy
  - Heat therapy
    - Causes vasodilation.
    - Improves blood flow.
    - Brings oxygen, nutrients, and leukocytes to the area.
    - Reduces pain.
    - Decreases edema.
    - Promotes muscle relaxation.
    - Decreases joint stiffness.
    - Applied with moist heat through compresses, soaks, or baths, or dry heat through electric heating pads, disposable hot packs, or aquathermia pads.
    - Precautions: do not use in areas that are bleeding, because bleeding could increase, or near abscesses, because heat could cause them to rupture. Use with caution in patients with sensory changes, neuropathies, or altered levels of consciousness, because they might not be able to sense that the temperature is too hot.

- Cold therapy
  - Causes vasoconstriction.
  - Reduces oxygen demands of the tissue.
  - Decreases pain.
  - Decreases swelling, decreases blood flow.
  - Prevents edema.
  - Provides anesthesia.
  - Relieves muscle spasm.
  - Applied through ice bags, cool compresses, cool soaks or baths, or with aquathermia pads.
  - Precautions: use with caution in patients that have edema because reabsorption slows. Do not use in areas that have impaired circulation, because cold will cause vasoconstriction. Use with caution in patients with sensory changes, neuropathies, or altered levels of consciousness, because they might not be able to sense that the temperature is too cold or that numbness is occurring.
- Caution is used when applying hot or cold therapy in patients with reduced ability to sense hot or cold as serious injury may occur, such as burns or circulatory problems.

For additional information on wound care, consult the following:

Ignatavicius DD, Workman ML, Rebar CR: *Medical-surgical nursing: patient-centered collaborative care,* ed 9, St. Louis, 2018, Elsevier.

Jarvis C: *Physical examination and health assessment,* ed 8, St. Louis, 2020, Elsevier.

Lewis SL, Bucher L, Heitkemper MM, et al: *Medical-surgical nursing,* ed 10, St. Louis, 2017, Elsevier.

Perry AG, Potter PA, Ostendorf WR: *Clinical nursing skills and techniques,* ed 9, St. Louis, 2018, Elsevier.

Potter PA, Perry AG, Stockert PA, Hall AM: *Fundamentals of nursing,* ed 10, St. Louis, 2021, Elsevier.

Yoost BL, Crawford LR: *Fundamentals of nursing: active learning for collaborative practice,* ed 2, St. Louis, 2020, Elsevier.

CHAPTER 25

Oxygen Administration

PULMONARY FUNCTION TESTS
- Forced vital capacity (FVC) measures the volume of air the patient can forcefully expire after the maximum amount of air is breathed in. The normal amount is approximately 4 L.
- Forced expiratory volume in one second (FEV_1) measures the volume of air expired in one second from the beginning of the FVC. The expected finding is 75% to 85% of FVC.
- Forced expiratory flow (FEF) measures the maximal flow rate reached during the middle of the FVC. Results are dependent on body size.
- Residual volume (RV) is the amount of air remaining in the lungs after forced expiration. The expected result is approximately 1 L.
- Functional residual capacity (FRC) is the volume of air that remains in the patient's lung after normal expiration. The predicted volume is 2.3 L.

OXYGEN THERAPY
- Oxygen is considered a drug; therefore a physician's order is required.
- Follow the Six Rights of Medication Administration when administering oxygen.

Nasal Cannula

- Place the prongs into the nares with the curved side on top.
- Loop the tubing over the patient's ear. Gauze or special tubing covers may be used as a cushion to prevent pressure areas.
- Tuck the tubing under the patient's chin and secure it with the sliding piece.
- Flow rates are:
  - 1 L/min = 24% O_2
  - 2 L/min = 28% O_2
  - 3 L/min = 32% O_2
  - 4 L/min = 36% O_2
  - 5 L/min = 40% O_2
  - 6 L/min = 44% O_2
- If patient requires more oxygen than 6 L of O_2, a mask may be needed.

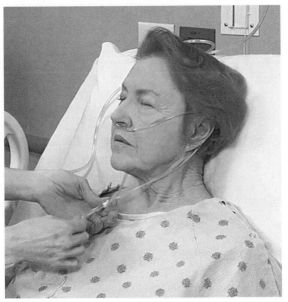

Nasal cannula. (From *Mosby's nursing video skills: basic, intermediate, and advanced skills*, ed 4, St. Louis, 2014, Elsevier.)

- Humidification may be added for comfort or for levels 4 L/min or higher.

Simple Face Mask

- Place the mask over the patient's mouth and nose.
- Secure the mask with the adjustable strap.
- Pinch the nose piece to ensure fit.
- Flow rates:
  - 5 L/min = 40% O_2
  - 6 L/min = 45% O_2
  - 7 L/min = 50% O_2
  - 8 L/min = 55% O_2
  - >8 L/min = 60% O_2
- Always humidify oxygen administered by mask.

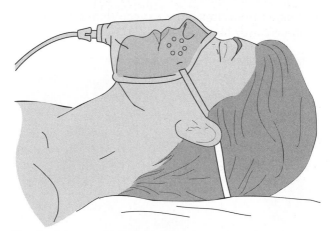

Simple face mask. (From Sorrentino SA, Remmert LN: *Mosby's textbook for nursing assistants,* ed 9, St. Louis, 2017, Elsevier.)

Partial Rebreather Mask

- Partial rebreather masks have a reservoir bag.
- Make sure the reservoir bag is filled before placing the mask on the patient.

- Flow Rates:
  - 6 to 15 L/min = 70% to 90% O_2
- Level of O_2 will depend on patient's overall respiratory and health status.
- Partial rebreather mask allows some of the exhaled air to enter the reservoir bag, which the patient rebreathes. The exhaled air contains carbon dioxide, which acts as a stimulus to breathe for some patients.
- Should not be run below 5 L/min. Reservoir bag should never be fully collapsed.

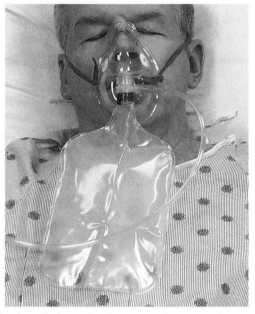

Partial rebreather mask with reservoir. (Copyright © Mosby's Clinical Skills: Essentials Collection.)

Nonrebreather Mask
- Nonrebreather masks have a reservoir bag.
- Make sure the reservoir bag is filled before placing the mask on the patient.
- Flow rates:
  - 10 to 15 L/min = 60% to 100% O_2
- The nonrebreather mask looks like a partial rebreather mask. The difference is that the nonrebreather mask has a one-way valve that prevents expired air from entering the reservoir bag.
- Reservoir bag should never be fully collapsed.

Venturi Mask
- Delivers the most accurate concentration of oxygen.
- Flow rates:
  - 4 to 12 L/min = 24% to 60% O_2
- The Venturi mask includes either a dial or a set of color-coded adapters. Each adaptor corresponds with a L/min setting to administer the correct percentage of oxygen.

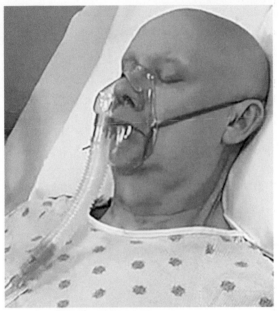

Venturi mask. (Copyright © Mosby's Clinical Skills: Essentials Collection.)

Trach Mask

- Patients with tracheostomies require a special mask and collar for oxygen administration.
- Oxygen for tracheostomies is always humidified.
- The mask is centered over the tracheostomy and secured around the neck with straps.
- Flow rates are similar to those of a simple face mask.

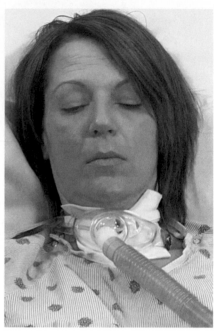

Trach mask and collar. (Copyright © Mosby's Clinical Skills: Essentials Collection)

Face Tent
- Delivers humidified oxygen at varied flow rates.
- Tent is centered over the face covering from the jaw upward.
- Secured with straps similar to face masks.

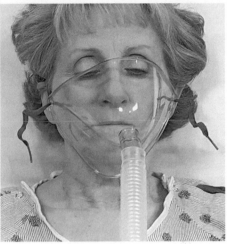

Face tent. (Copyright © Mosby's Clinical Skills: Essentials Collection)

COMMON LUNG DISORDERS
Asthma
- **Signs and symptoms:** Dyspnea, cough, tachypnea
- **Listen for:** Decreased sounds with wheezes

Atelectasis
- **Signs and symptoms:** Tachypnea, cyanosis, use of accessory muscles
- **Listen for:** Decreased sound with crackles or absent sounds over a lung field

Bronchiectasis
- **Signs and symptoms:** Chronic cough with large amounts of foul-smelling sputum production, coughing up blood, cough worsened by lying on one side, fatigue, shortness of breath worsened by

exercise, weight loss, wheezing, paleness, bluish skin discoloration, and breath odor; clubbing of fingers may be present
- **Listen for:** Wheezes and crackles

Bronchitis
- **Signs and symptoms:** Cough with sputum, sore throat and fever, prolonged expiration
- **Listen for:** Prolonged expiration, wheezes, crackles

Emphysema
- **Signs and symptoms:** Dyspnea, cough with sputum
- **Listen for:** Wheezes, rhonchi

Neoplasm
- **Signs and symptoms:** Cough with sputum, chest pain
- **Listen for:** Decreased breath sounds

Pleural Effusion
- **Signs and symptoms:** Pain, dyspnea, pallor, fever, cough
- **Listen for:** Decreased breath sounds, friction rub

Pneumonia
- **Signs and symptoms:** Chills, productive cough
- **Listen for:** Fine crackles or friction rub

Pneumothorax
- **Signs and symptoms:** Pain, dyspnea, cyanosis, tachypnea
- **Listen for:** Decreased sound on affected side

Pulmonary Edema

- **Signs and symptoms:** Tachypnea, cough, cyanosis, orthopnea, use of accessory muscles
- **Listen for:** Rales, rhonchi, wheezes

For additional information on oxygen administration, consult the following:

Ignatavicius DD, Workman ML, Rebar CR: *Medical-surgical nursing: patient-centered collaborative care*, ed 9, St. Louis, 2018, Elsevier.

Lewis SL, Bucher L, Heitkemper MM, et al: *Medical-surgical nursing*, ed 10, St. Louis, 2017, Elsevier.

Perry AG, Potter PA, Ostendorf WR: *Clinical nursing skills and techniques*, ed 9, St. Louis, 2018, Elsevier.

Potter PA, Perry AG, Stockert PA, Hall AM: *Fundamentals of nursing*, ed 10, St. Louis, 2021, Elsevier.

Yoost BL, Crawford LR: *Fundamentals of nursing: active learning for collaborative practice*, ed 2, St. Louis, 2020, Elsevier.

CHAPTER 26

Nutrition and Diets

ESSENTIAL COMPONENTS OF THE DIGESTIVE SYSTEM

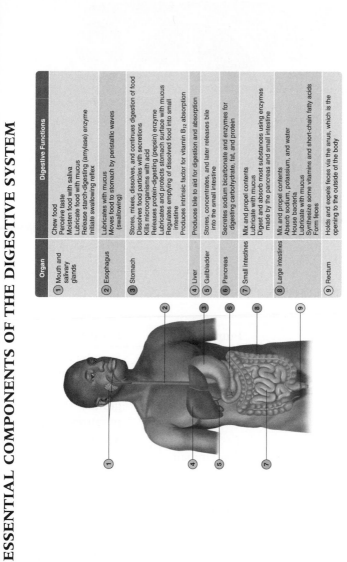

Organ	Digestive Functions
① Mouth and salivary glands	Chew food Perceive taste Moisten food with saliva Lubricate food with mucus Release starch-digesting (amylase) enzyme Initiate swallowing reflex
② Esophagus	Lubricates with mucus Moves food to stomach by peristaltic waves (swallowing)
③ Stomach	Stores, mixes, dissolves, and continues digestion of food Dissolves food particles with secretions Kills microorganisms with acid Releases protein-digesting (pepsin) enzyme Lubricates and protects stomach surface with mucus Regulates emptying of dissolved food into small intestine Produces intrinsic factor for vitamin B_{12} absorption
④ Liver	Produces bile to aid for digestion and absorption
⑤ Gallbladder	Stores, concentrates, and later releases bile into the small intestine
⑥ Pancreas	Secretes sodium bicarbonate and enzymes for digesting carbohydrate, fat, and protein
⑦ Small intestines	Mix and propel contents Lubricate with mucus Digest and absorb most substances using enzymes made by the pancreas and small intestine
⑧ Large intestines	Mix and propel contents Absorb sodium, potassium, and water House bacteria Lubricate with mucus Synthesize some vitamins and short-chain fatty acids Form feces
⑨ Rectum	Holds and expels feces via the anus, which is the opening to the outside of the body

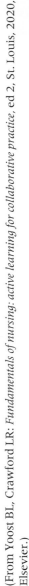

(From Yoost BL, Crawford LR: *Fundamentals of nursing: active learning for collaborative practice*, ed 2, St. Louis, 2020, Elsevier.)

MY PLATE RECOMMENDATIONS

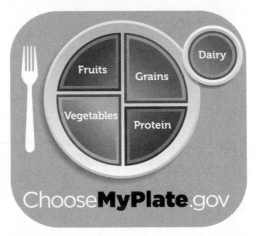

(From U.S. Department of Agriculture: Dietary Guidelines for Americans, 2018. Retrieved from www.choosemyplate. gov/Myplate.)

NUTRIENTS

Type	Function	Food Sources
Carbohydrate	Energy, body temperature	Simple: sugars, fruits, nuts Complex: grains, potatoes, milk
Protein	Tissue growth, tissue repair	Meat, fish, eggs, milk, poultry, beans, peas, nuts
Fat	Energy and repair, carries vitamins A and D	Animal fat, meat, nuts, milk, dairy products, fish, poultry

NUTRIENTS—Cont'd

Type	Function	Food Sources
Water	Carries nutrients, regulates body processes, lubricates joints	Liquids, most fruits and vegetables

VITAMINS

Type	Function	Food Sources
A (retinol)	Helps eyes, skin, hair, bones, and teeth; fights infection	Yellow fruits and vegetables, liver, kidney, fish
B_1 (thiamine)	Maintains nerves, aids carbohydrate function	Bread, cereal, beans, peas, pork, liver, eggs, milk
B_2 (riboflavin)	Maintains skin, mouth, nerve functions, metabolism of protein	Dairy, cheese, eggs, cereal, dark green vegetables, whole grains
B_3 (niacin)	Oxidation of proteins and carbohydrates, formation of fatty acids	Meat, fish, poultry, eggs, nuts, bread, cereal, dried beans, whole grains
B_5 (pantothenic acid)	Metabolism of carbohydrates, fats, and proteins	Whole grain cereals, potatoes, legumes, broccoli

Continued

VITAMINS—Cont'd

Type	Function	Food Sources
B_6 (pyridoxine)	Synthesis of amino acids	Spinach, squash, bell peppers
B_7 Biotin	Enables formation of DNA and RNA	Liver, legumes, tomatoes, egg yolk
B_9 (folic acid)	Synthesis of DNA, red blood cell formation, rapidly growing cells	Green vegetables, oranges, strawberries, dried beans, peas/nuts, enriched breads
B_{12} (cyanocobalamin)	Aids muscles, nerves, heart, metabolism	Organ meats, milk
C (ascorbic acid)	Maintains integrity of cells, repairs tissue, synthesizes collagen	Citrus fruits, tomatoes, green vegetables, potatoes
D	Enables body to use calcium and phosphorus	Dairy, margarine, fish, liver, eggs
F	Antioxidant, protects immune system	Peanuts, vegetable oils
K	Aids in blood clotting	Dark green leafy vegetables

MINERALS

Calcium	Renews bones and teeth, regulates heart and nerves	Milk, green vegetables, cheese, salmon, legumes
Phosphorus	Renews bones and teeth, maintains nerve function	Cheese, oats, meat, milk, fish, poultry, nuts
Iron	Renews hemoglobin	Meat, eggs, liver, flour, yellow or green vegetables
Iodine	Regulates thyroid	Table salt, seafood
Magnesium	Component of enzymes	Grains, green vegetables
Sodium	Maintains water balance, nerve function	Salt, cured meats
Potassium	Maintains nerve function	Meat, milk, vegetables
Chloride	Formation of gastric juices	Salt
Zinc	Component of enzymes	Meat, seafood

ASSISTANCE WITH FEEDING AN ADULT

- Follow any dietary and nutritional orders, including food texture and use of thickening agents.
- Avoid rushing to prevent aspiration.

- May delegate feeding to unlicensed assistive personnel (UAP) if UAP is instructed in proper techniques and dietary restrictions.
- Provide oral care before and after feeding.
  - If the patient has dentures, ensure that they are in place and well fitted.
- Elevate the patient's head at least 30 to 45 degrees unless contraindicated.
  - Special caution should be taken if the patient has impaired swallowing.
  - If the patient has one-sided muscle weakness, have the patient turn the head to the affected side to assist in airway protection.
  - Chin-tucking may help to prevent aspiration.
- If assistive devices are in use, follow the occupational or nutrition therapy guidelines or the manufacturer's instructions for use.
- Allow at least 30 minutes for each meal.
  - Offer small bites (1/2 to 1 teaspoon).
  - Wait at least 10 seconds between bites.
- Alternate food with fluids.
- Avoid unnecessary use of straws to prevent air ingestion.
- Observe for the rise and fall of the patient's larynx to verify swallowing.
- Check the patient's mouth frequently to prevent retention of food in the cheeks (pocketing).

TYPES OF DIETS

Type	Description	Patient Condition
Regular	All essential nutrients, without restriction	No special diet required

TYPES OF DIETS—Cont'd

Type	Description	Patient Condition
Clear liquid	Clear broth, tea, clear soda, juices without pulp, popsicles, and gelatin	Preoperative or postoperative, gastrointestinal problems, or before some diagnostic testing
Full liquid	Milk and milk products, yogurt, strained cream soups, liquid dietary supplements, and juice with pulp	In transition from clear to regular diet, inability to tolerate solid food
Thickened liquids	Commercial thickening agents added to liquid; no nuts, seeds, hard, or raw foods	Difficulty swallowing and risk for aspiration
Pureed	Foods placed in a blender into a pulplike consistency; no raw eggs, nuts, or seeds	Inability to safely chew or swallow solid food
Mechanical soft	Regular diet chopped or ground	Difficulty chewing or swallowing
Soft	Soft consistency and mild spice	Difficulty swallowing or recovering from gastrointestinal problems

Continued

TYPES OF DIETS—Cont'd

Type	Description	Patient Condition
Bland	No spicy food	Ulcers or colitis
Low residue	No bulky foods, apples, or nuts	Colorectal disease
High calorie	High protein, vitamins, and fat	Malnourished
Low calorie	Decreased fat, no whole milk, cream, eggs, complex carbohydrates	Overweight/obesity
Diabetic (ADA)	Balance of protein, carbohydrates, fat	Insulin-food imbalance
High protein	Meat, fish, milk, cheese, poultry, eggs	Tissue repair, underweight
Low fat	Limited butter, cream, whole milk, and eggs	Gallbladder, liver, or heart disease
Low cholesterol	Limited meat and cheese	Need for decreased fat intake
Low sodium	Limited soups, processed foods, pickles, and lunch meat	Heart or renal disease
Salt free	No salt	Heart or renal disease
Tube feeding	Formulas or liquid	Oral surgery, oral or esophageal cancers, inability to eat and/or swallow

TOTAL PARENTERAL NUTRITION (TPN)

- TPN may be administered through a peripherally inserted central catheter (PICC) line or central venous catheter (CVC) using an infusion pump.
- Infusions with greater than 10% dextrose concentration typically require a CVC rather than a peripheral intravenous site.
- TPN may be prescribed for patients who:
  - Do not have a functioning gastrointestinal (GI) tract, or
  - are unable to ingest, digest, or absorb essential nutrients due to conditions, such as some stages of Crohn's disease or ulcerative gastritis, gastrointestinal obstruction, diarrhea unresponsive to treatment, abdominal trauma, burns, or postoperative status.
- Monitor
  - Weight
  - Blood glucose levels (q6h or more frequently until stabilized)
  - Complete blood count (CBC)
  - Electrolytes
  - Blood urea nitrogen (BUN)
  - Fluid intake and output
- Maintenance
  - Tubing should be marked and clearly identified so that no other solution is infused through it.
  - Tubing should be changed every 24 hours, with aseptic technique used to minimize the risk of contamination
  - Site dressing should be changed every 48 hours, with assessment for signs and symptoms of infection (redness, swelling, or drainage)
- Potential complications
  - Site infections

- Air embolism
- Catheter-related infections
- Dislodgment or occlusion of tubing
- Metabolic complications

For additional information on nutrition and diets, consult the following:

Potter PA, Perry AG, Stockert PA, Hall AM: *Fundamentals of nursing*, ed 10, St. Louis, 2021, Elsevier.

Schlenker E, Gilbert J: *Williams' essentials of nutrition and diet therapy,* ed 12, St. Louis, 2018, Elsevier.

Yoost BL, Crawford LR: *Fundamentals of nursing: active learning for collaborative practice*, ed 2, St. Louis, 2020, Elsevier.

CHAPTER 27

Diagnostic Testing and Procedures

SPECIMEN COLLECTION
Blood Collection Tubes
- **Yellow:** Used for blood cultures
- **Light blue/citrate:** Used for coagulation studies: PT, PTT, and fibrinogen
- **Red:** Used for most blood chemistries and serology tests and blood bank testing
- **Red/black:** Used for most blood chemistries and serology tests
- **Green:** Used for stat blood chemistries
- **Lavender/purple/navy:** Used for hematology studies
- **Gray:** Used for glucose, blood alcohol levels, and lactic acid

Culture and Sensitivity Specimen Collection

Type of Specimen	Collection Device	Specimen Collection and Transport (always use proper standard precautions and PPE when collecting specimens, label all specimens, and transport according to facility policy)
Wound culture	Sterile cotton-tipped swab culturette or syringe	Cleanse wound with sterile saline. Moisten swab with sterile saline. Insert the swab into draining tissue and cover it with drainage. Reinsert the swab into the culturette tube making sure nothing touches the swab. Close the tube and crush the ampule of collection medium within the tube if required.
Blood culture	Two culture media tubes, one for aerobic culture and one for anaerobic culture. Amount of blood needed varies	Cleanse the venipuncture site with antiseptic per facility policy and allow it to dry. Perform venipuncture. Collect blood in culture tubes.

Continued

Culture and Sensitivity Specimen Collection—Cont'd

Type of Specimen	Collection Device	Specimen Collection and Transport (always use proper standard precautions and PPE when collecting specimens, label all specimens, and transport according to facility policy)
Stool Culture	Clean cup with seal top (not necessary to be sterile) and tongue blade; small amount needed about the size of a walnut, or several mL of liquid feces	Have the patient defecate into a clean bedpan or collection hat. Use a clean tongue blade to collect feces and transfer it to a collection container without touching the outside surface. Secure the top of the container.
Urine culture	Syringe and sterile cup: 1-5 mL of urine	Use syringe to collect specimen from the needleless collection port if patient has Foley catheter. Have patient follow procedure to obtain clean-voided specimen if not catheterized. Transfer urine into sterile container by injecting urine from syringe or pouring it from the collection container.

Agency policies may differ on type of containers, amount of specimen material required, and bagging.
Adapted from Potter PA, Perry AG, Stockert PA, Hall A: *Fundamentals of nursing*, ed 9, St. Louis, 2017, Elsevier.

LABORATORY TESTS: BLOOD
Complete Blood Count (CBC)

Blood Component	Normal Values*
Red blood cells (RBCs)	Males: $4.7\text{-}6.1 \times 10^6$ mcL
	Females: $4.2\text{-}5.4 \times 10^6$ mcL
White blood cells (WBCs)	$5000\text{-}10,000/\text{mm}^3$
Neutrophils	Adult: 55%-70%
	Child: 30%-60%
Lymphocytes	Adult: 20%-40%
	Child: 25%-50%
Monocytes	2%-8%
Eosinophils	1%-4%
Basophils	0.5%-1%
Hemoglobin (Hgb)	Males: 14-18 g/dL
	Females: 12-16 g/dL
Hematocrit (Hct)	Males: 42%-52%
	Females: 37%-47%
Platelets	$150,000\text{-}400,000/\text{mm}^3$

*Ranges may vary by facility.

Coagulation Studies

Coagulation Test	Normal Values*
Platelet	$150,000\text{-}400,000/\text{mm}^3$
International normalized ratio (INR)	0.8-1.1

Coagulation Studies—Cont'd

Coagulation Test	Normal Values
Prothrombin time (PT)	11-12.5 sec
Partial thromboplastin time (PTT)	60-70 sec
Partial thromboplastin time, activated (aPTT)	30-40 sec

*Ranges may vary by facility.

Basic Metabolic Panel

Blood Chemistry	Normal Values*
Sodium (Na^+)	136-145 mEq/L
Potassium (K^+)	3.5-5 mEq/L
Chloride (Cl^-)	98-106 mEq/L
Carbon dioxide (CO_2)	23-30 mEq/L
Blood urea nitrogen (BUN)	10-20 mg/dL
Creatinine (Cr)	Males: 0.6-1.2 mg/dL
	Females: 0.5-1.1 mg/dL
Glucose	74–106 mg/dL

*Ranges may vary by facility.

Other Electrolytes

Electrolyte	Normal Values*
Calcium (Ca++)	9-10.5 mg/dL
Magnesium (Mg)	1.3-2.1 mg/dL
Phosphorus	3-4.5 mg/dL

*Ranges may vary by facility.

Common Electrolyte Imbalances

- Hyponatremia (less than 136 mEq/L)
  - **Signs and symptoms:** Fatigue, confusion, abdominal cramps, diarrhea, nausea, weakness, seizures
  - **Causes:** Water intoxication, kidney disease, vomiting, diarrhea, excessive use of hypotonic saline IV solutions, syndrome of inappropriate antidiuretic hormone secretion (SIADH)
  - **Interventions:** Monitor vital signs, intake and output (I & O), and laboratory results; increase sodium intake; restrict water; administer hypertonic saline IV solutions as ordered
- Hypernatremia (greater than 145 mEq/L)
  - **Signs and symptoms:** Thirst; dry, sticky mucous membranes; dry tongue and skin; flushed skin; increased temperature; weakness; confusion; irritability; decreased level of consciousness
  - **Causes:** Excessive sodium intake, hypertonic saline IV solutions, excessive loss of water, diabetes insipidus
  - **Interventions:** Monitor vital signs, I & O, level of consciousness, and laboratory results; limit salt intake; increase water intake; administer hypotonic saline IV solutions as ordered
- Hypokalemia (less than 3.5 mEq/L)
  - **Signs and symptoms:** Weakness, fatigue, anorexia, abdominal distention, arrhythmias, decreased bowel sounds
  - **Causes:** Diarrhea, potassium-wasting diuretics, inadequate intake
  - **Interventions:** Monitor heart rate and rhythm, monitor laboratory results, increase potassium intake through foods, oral supplements, or in maintenance IVs. *Never administer potassium IV push.*

- Hyperkalemia (greater than 5 mEq/L)
  - **Signs and symptoms:** Anxiety, arrhythmias, confusion, increased bowel sounds, paralysis, paresthesia
  - **Causes:** Burns, renal failure, potassium-sparing diuretics, acidosis
  - **Interventions:** Monitor heart rate and rhythm; monitor laboratory results; limit potassium intake through foods, oral supplements, or in maintenance IVs.
- Hypocalcemia (less than 9 mEq/L)
  - **Signs and symptoms:** Abdominal cramps, tingling, muscle spasms, convulsions, dysrhythmias
  - **Causes:** Parathyroid dysfunction, vitamin D deficiency, pancreatitis, inadequate intake, chronic alcoholism
  - **Interventions:** Monitor heart rate and rhythm, administer calcium as ordered, begin seizure precautions
- Hypercalcemia (greater than 10.5 mEq/L)
  - **Signs and symptoms:** Lethargy, coma, decreased muscle strength and tone, anorexia, nausea, vomiting, constipation, pathologic fractures, dysrhythmias
  - **Causes:** Hyperparathyroidism, bone cancer or metastasis, osteoporosis, prolonged bed rest
  - **Interventions:** Monitor heart rate and rhythm, increase fluids, increase activity
- Hypomagnesemia (less than 1.3 mEq/L)
  - **Signs and symptoms:** Hyperactive deep tendon reflexes, irritable nerves, seizures, tachyarrhythmias, altered level of consciousness, dysphagia, nausea, vomiting
  - **Causes:** Prolonged diarrhea, laxative abuse, Crohn's or colitis, polyuria, decreased intake or absorption

- **Interventions:** Assess vital signs, mental status, and swallowing; monitor potassium, calcium, and magnesium levels; institute seizure precautions; administer supplements as ordered
- Hypermagnesemia (greater than 2.1 mEq/L)
  - **Signs and symptoms:** Lethargy, respiratory difficulty, coma, nausea, vomiting, decreased deep tendon reflexes and muscle strength, hypotension, dysrhythmias
  - **Causes:** Excessive intake, prolonged intake in IV or TPN, renal failure, adrenal insufficiency
  - **Interventions:** Assess vital signs, neuromuscular status, and mental status; encourage fluids; provide respiratory support as needed
- Hypochloremia (less than 98 mEq/L)
  - **Signs and symptoms:** Fatigue, dizziness, hypotension, irritable nerves
  - **Causes:** Loss of fluid, severe vomiting or diarrhea, prolonged diuretic or laxative use, SIADH
  - **Interventions:** Monitor vital signs, I & O, and laboratory results
- Hyperchloremia (greater than 106 mEq/L)
  - **Signs and symptoms:** Thirst; dry mucous membranes, tongue, and skin; lethargy; deep breathing
  - **Causes:** High sodium level, kidney failure, diabetes insipidus, diabetic coma
  - **Interventions:** Monitor vital signs, I & O, level of consciousness, and laboratory results; limit salt intake; increase water intake; administer hypotonic saline IV solutions as ordered
- Hypophosphatemia (less than 3 mEq/L)
  - **Signs and symptoms:** Weakness, bone and joint pain, decreased deep tendon reflexes, weak pulse, shallow respirations,

- **Causes:** Lack of vitamin D, hypocalcemia, hyperglycemia, hyperventilation, respiratory alkalosis, chronic diarrhea, laxative use
- **Interventions:** Assess vital signs and muscle strength, administer phosphorus as ordered
- Hyperphosphatemia (greater than 4.5 mEq/L)
  - **Signs and symptoms:** Abdominal cramps, numbness and tingling, tachycardia, nausea, diarrhea
  - **Causes:** Kidney failure, hypoparathyroidism, acid-base imbalances
  - **Interventions:** Monitor vital signs and I & O; monitor phosphorus and calcium levels, blood urea nitrogen (BUN), and creatinine; avoid phosphorus-rich foods

Hemoglobin A1C (Hb A$_{1c}$, glycosylated hemoglobin)
- Normal values:
  - Nondiabetic: 4%–5.9%
  - Diabetic in good control: <7%
  - Diabetic in far control: 8%–9%
  - Diabetic in poor control: >9%
- Used to test blood sugar level over a period of 2 to 3 months.

Kidney Function Tests
- Blood urea nitrogen (BUN) (see Blood Chemistries table for values)
  - Elevated BUN may indicate: decreased renal glomerular function, a high-protein diet, or dehydration.
- Creatinine (see Blood Chemistries table for values)
  - Elevated in renal impairment.
- Estimated glomerular filtration rate (eGFR)
  - Glomerular filtration rate measures kidney function and the severity of kidney disease.
  - Creatinine level, age, gender, and ethnicity are used in a formula to estimate the GFR.

- Levels less than 60 mL/min/2.73m^2 show mild to moderate loss of kidney function.
- A level less than 15 mL/min/2.73m^2 indicates kidney failure.

Liver Function Tests

Test	Normal Value*
Aspartate aminotransferase (AST)	0-35 U/L
Alanine aminotransferase (ALT)	4-36 U/L
Alkaline phosphatase (ALP)	Adult: 30-120 U/L
Bilirubin: direct	0.1-0.3 mg/dL
Bilirubin: total	0.3-1.0 mg/dL
Amylase	30-220 U/L
Lipase	0-160 U/L

*Ranges may vary by facility.

Lipid Profile

Component	Normal Value*
Cholesterol	<200 mg/dL
Low-density lipoprotein (LDL)	<130 mg/dL
High-density lipoprotein (HDL)	Male: >45 mg/dL Female: >55 mg/dL
Triglycerides	Male: 40-160 mg/dL Female: 35-135 mg/dL

*Ranges may vary by facility.

Cardiac Function Tests

Creatine phosphokinase (CK)	Levels rise 6 hr after an acute myocardial infarction (MI), peaking at 18 hr and returning to baseline within 3 days Normal: Male 55-170 U/L; Female 30-135 U/L
CK-MB isoenzyme	Increases 4 hr after an acute MI; peaks in 18 hr; remains elevated for up to 48 hr Normal: <0%
Troponin T	Increases 4-6 hr after an MI; peaks at 10-24 hr; the elevation can last 10 days Normal: <0.1 ng/mL
Troponin I	Increases 4-6 hr after an MI; peaks at 10-24 hr; the increase lasts up to 4 days Normal: <0.03ng/mL
Myoglobin	Rises within 3 hr of MI; peaks at 8–12 hrs; returns to normal in 24 hrs Normal: <90 mcg/L
Brain natriuretic peptides	Identifies patients with heart failure Normal: <100 pg/mL Heart failure likely >400 pg/mL

Ranges may vary per facility.

Arterial Blood Gases (ABGs)

- Help to evaluate respiratory function and determine acid-base balance.
- Interpretation of arterial blood gas requires a systematic approach, using the following normal values:

pH	7.35-7.45
Pa_{CO_2}	35-45 mm Hg
HCO_3^-	21-28 mEq/L
PaO_2	80-100 mm Hg
O_2 saturation	95%-100%

- Step 1: examine the oxygenation status by examining the PaO_2 and O_2 saturation values.
  - PaO_2 of 60 to 80 mm Hg: mild hypoxemia.
  - PaO_2 of 40 to 60 mm Hg: moderate hypoxemia.
  - PaO_2 less than 40 mm Hg: severe hypoxemia.
- Step 2: Examine the pH and determine whether the value falls within the normal range.
  - pH less than 7.35, underlying acidosis.
  - pH greater than 7.45, underlying alkalosis.
  - Normal pH may indicate that compensation has occurred.
- Step 3: Examine the Pa_{CO_2} and HCO_3^- values to determine whether the underlying disorder is metabolic or respiratory.
  - Pa_{CO_2} is abnormal and the HCO_3^- is normal, then there is a respiratory imbalance. In respiratory disorders, there is an inverse relationship between the pH and the Pa_{CO_2} values.
  - Pa_{CO_2} is normal and the HCO_3^- is abnormal, then there is a metabolic disorder.

Acid-Base Imbalance	pH	Paco$_2$	HCO$_3^-$
Respiratory acidosis	↓	↑	Normal
Respiratory alkalosis	↑	↓	Normal
Metabolic acidosis	↓	Normal	↓
Metabolic alkalosis	↑	Normal	↑

↓, Decreased value; ↑, increased value.

From Yoost BL, Crawford LR: *Fundamentals of nursing: active learning for collaborative practice,* ed 2, St. Louis, 2020, Elsevier.

- Step 4: Interpret ABGs to determine whether compensation is occurring.
  - When an acid-base imbalance occurs the body tries to compensate to keep the pH in normal range.
  - The Paco$_2$ or HCO$_3^-$ will increase or decrease, depending on the imbalance, to attempt to keep the pH within normal range.

Acid-Base Imbalance	pH	Paco$_2$	HCO$_3^-$
Compensated respiratory acidosis	On the ↓ side of normal	↑	↑
Compensated respiratory alkalosis	On the ↑ side of normal	↓	↓
Compensated metabolic acidosis	On the ↓ side of normal	↓	↓
Compensated metabolic alkalosis	On the ↑ side of normal	↑	↑

↓, Decreased value; ↑, increased value.

From Yoost BL, Crawford LR: *Fundamentals of nursing: active learning for collaborative practice,* ed 2, St. Louis, 2020, Elsevier.

Therapeutic Drug Monitoring
- Some medications are monitored with serum drug levels.
- Therapeutic levels and toxic levels have been determined for many drugs.
- Peak and trough drug levels may be drawn when a steady concentration of the medication is needed for treatment.

Common medications monitored through serum levels:

Medication	Classification	Therapeutic Level*	Toxic Level*
Gentamycin	Antibiotic	5-10 mcg/mL	>12 mcg/mL
Vancomycin	Antibiotic	10-25 mcg/mL	>30 mcg/mL
Carbamazepine	Anticonvulsant	5-12 mcg/mL	>12 mcg/mL
Phenobarbital	Anticonvulsant	10-30 mcg/mL	>40 mcg/mL
Phenytoin	Anticonvulsant	10-20 mcg/mL	>30 mcg/mL
Valproic acid	Anticonvulsant	50-100 mcg/mL	>100 mcg/mL
Amitriptyline	Antidepressant	120-150 ng/mL	>500 ng/mL
Lithium	Antimanic	0.8-1.2 mEq/L	>2 mEq/L
Digoxin	Antiarrhythmic	0.8-2 ng/mL	>2.4 ng/mL
Theophylline	Bronchodilator	10-20 mcg/mL	>20 mcg/mL

*Levels may vary by facility.

Adapted from Pagana KD, Pagana TJ: *Mosby's manual of diagnostic and laboratory tests*, ed 6, St. Louis, 2018, Elsevier.

LABORATORY TESTS: URINE
Urinalysis

Component	Normal Value	Abnormal Values
Color	Light yellow to amber	Dark yellow to amber: • Concentrated urine • Presence of bilirubin Blue/green: • Pseudomonal urinary tract infection Light straw/very pale yellow: • Alcohol ingestion • High fluid intake • Dilute urine Orange: • Presence of bile • Fever • Several drugs known to alter the color of urine
Clarity	Clear to slightly hazy	Cloudy: may indicate bacteria and red or white blood cells
Specific gravity	1.005-1.030	Increased: • Acute glomerulonephritis • Congestive heart failure • Dehydration • Diabetes mellitus • Low fluid intake • Liver failure • Vomiting and diarrhea

Continued

LABORATORY TESTS: URINE—Cont'd

Component	Normal Value	Abnormal Values
		Decreased: • Antidiuretic hormone deficiency • Chronic pyelonephritis • Diuretics • High fluid intake
Potential hydrogen (pH)	4.6-8.0	Increased: • Bacteriuria • Chronic renal failure • Metabolic alkalosis • Urinary tract infection • Starvation Decreased: • Dehydration • Diabetes mellitus • Diarrhea • Fever • Urinary tract infection
Glucose	Negative	Increased: • Diabetes mellitus • Infection • Stress
Ketones	Negative	Increased: • Alcoholism • Anorexia • Diabetes mellitus • Diarrhea • Fasting • Fever • High-protein diet • Postanesthesia • Starvation • Vomiting

LABORATORY TESTS: URINE—Cont'd

Component	Normal Value	Abnormal Values
Red blood cells	≤2	Increased: • Acute tubular necrosis • Benign prostatic hypertrophy • Renal calculi • Hemophilia • Renal trauma • Urinary tract infection • Menstruation
Protein	0-8 mg/dL	Increased: • Diabetes mellitus • Emotional stress • Exercise • Glomerulonephritis • Pyelonephritis
Bilirubin	Negative	Increased: • Cirrhosis of the liver • Hepatitis • Obstructive jaundice
Bacteria	Negative	Increased: • Urinary tract infection

Adapted from Pagana KD, Pagana TJ: *Mosby's manual of diagnostic and laboratory tests,* ed 6, St. Louis, 2018, Elsevier.

24-Hour Urine for Creatinine Clearance
• Urine is collected for 24 hours in a container that is kept on ice.
• The test begins after a patient voids, and the urine is discarded. Collection begins with the next void and urine is collected for 24 hours.
• A blood sample for creatinine is drawn.
• Creatinine is measured in both the 24-hour urine sample and in the blood sample.

- Test is performed when creatinine level or eGFR are abnormal.
- Used to detect acute kidney injury and chronic kidney disease.

LABORATORY TESTS: STOOL
- Stool samples are collected to test for occult blood, fat, urobilinogen levels, and ova and parasites.
- Fecal occult blood testing can detect very small amounts of blood in the stool.
- Bleeding can be anywhere along the gastrointestinal tract.
- Fecal occult blood testing is used in colorectal cancer screening along with sigmoidoscopy or colonoscopy.
- The presence of fecal fat or steatorrhea indicates an inability to digest dietary fat.
- Urobilinogen is produced by the breakdown of bilirubin.
- Normal urobilinogen: 50 to 300 mg/24 hours.
- Urobilinogen is increased as a result of red blood cell destruction. It is decreased as a result of biliary obstruction or in severe liver disease.

LABORATORY TESTS: CULTURE AND SENSITIVITY
- Specimens from blood, urine, stool, wounds, drainage, sputum, or the throat can be cultured and tested for bacteria.
- If bacteria are present, the specimen is exposed to various antibiotics to determine sensitivity or which antibiotic therapy would be most effective to treat the strain of bacteria.
- Testing will also determine which resistant bacteria continue to grow in the presence of certain antibiotics.

DIAGNOSTIC EXAMINATIONS

- **Angiography:** Records cardiac pressures, function, and output. Patient may need special postprocedure vital signs taken.
- **Arteriography:** Radiographic examination with injections of dye used to locate occlusion. Patient may need special postprocedure vital signs taken.
- **Arthrography:** Radiographic examination of the bones.
- **Arthroscopy:** Procedure that allows examination of the joint through a scope.
- **Barium study:** Radiographic examination to locate polyps, tumors, or other colon problems. Barium is instilled and needs to be passed in the stool after procedure.
- **Barium swallow:** Detects esophageal narrowing, varices, strictures, or tumors. Barium is swallowed and needs to be passed in the stool after procedure.
- **Biopsy:** Removal of specific tissue to detect cancer and other abnormalities. Assess patient for pain or bleeding after procedure.
- **Bone densitometry:** Test to determine bone mineral content and density; used to diagnose osteoporosis.
- **Bone marrow biopsy:** Examination of a piece of tissue from bone marrow. Assess patient for pain and bleeding after procedure.
- **Bone scan:** Radioisotope used to locate tumors or other bone disorders. Patient must be able to lie flat.
- **Brain scan:** Radioisotope used to locate tumors, strokes, or seizure disorders. Patient must be able to lie flat.
- **Bronchoscopy:** Inspection of the larynx, trachea, and bronchi with a flexible scope. Patient may need sedation. Be sure the swallowing reflex returns before offering fluids or food.

- **Cardiac catheterization:** Uses dye to visualize the heart's arteries. Patient may need special postprocedure vital signs taken.
- **Chest radiographs:** Xrays used to look for pneumonia, cancer, and other diseases of the lung.
- **Cholangiography:** Radiographic examination of the biliary ducts.
- **Cholecystography:** Radiographic examination of the gallbladder.
- **Colonoscopy:** Use of a flexible scope to view the colon. Patient will need a bowel preparation and will be sedated during the procedure.
- **Colposcopy:** Examination of the cervix and vagina.
- **Computed tomography (CT) scan:** Three-dimensional radiography. Patient must be able to lie flat.
- **Culdoscopy:** Flexible tube used to view the pelvic organs.
- **Cystoscopy:** Direct visualization of bladder with cystoscope.
- **Dilatation and curettage:** Dilatation of the cervix followed by endometrial cleansing done in surgery.
- **Doppler:** Ultrasonography used to show venous or arterial patency.
- **Echocardiography:** Ultrasonography that records the structure and functions of the heart.
- **Electrocardiography (EKG or ECG):** Records electrical impulses generated by the heart.
- **Electroencephalography (EEG):** Records electrical activity of the brain while the patient rests.
- **Electromyography (EMG):** Records electrical activity of the muscles.
- **Endoscopy:** Inspection of upper gastrointestinal (GI) tract with a flexible scope. Patient may need to

be sedated, and swallowing reflex may be diminished for a period of time after the procedure.

- **Endoscopic retrograde cholangiopancreatography (ERCP):** Radiographic examination of the gallbladder and pancreas.

- **Exercise stress test:** Recording of the heart rate, activity, and blood pressure while the body is at work.

- **Fluoroscopy:** Radiographic examination with pictures displayed on television monitor.

- **GI series:** Radiographic examination using barium to locate ulcers. Barium is swallowed and must be passed through the GI tract after the examination.

- **Glucose tolerance test (GTT):** Determines ability to tolerate an oral glucose load; used to establish diabetes.

- **Hemoccult:** Detects blood in stool, emesis, and elsewhere.

- **Holter monitor:** Checks and records irregular heart rates and rhythms generally over a 24-hour period or longer.

- **Intravenous pyelography (IVP):** Radiographic examination of the kidneys after dye injection.

- **KUB:** Radiographic examination of the kidneys, ureter, and bladder.

- **Laparoscopy:** Abdominal examination with a flexible scope, usually through a small incision in the abdomen or through the umbilicus.

- **Lumbar puncture:** Sampling of spinal fluid, often called a spinal tap. Can be done at bedside or in a special procedures room.

- **Magnetic resonance imaging (MRI):** Three-dimensional radiograph similar to CT scan except that magnets are used instead of radiation. Contraindicated in patients with metal in their bodies, such as some pacemakers, inner ear implants, or fragments of metal from gunshot wounds or industrial accidents.

- **Mammography:** Radiographic examination of the breast.
- **Myelography:** Injection of dye into the subarachnoid space to view brain and spinal cord.
- **Oximetry:** Method to monitor arterial blood saturation.
- **Pap smear:** Sample of cells from the cervix are examined. Detects cervical cancer.
- **Proctoscopy:** Inspection of lower colon with a flexible scope. Patient may need to be sedated.
- **Pulmonary function test (PFT):** Measures lung capacity and volume to detect respiratory problems.
- **Pyelography:** Radiographic examination of the kidneys.
- **Sigmoidoscopy:** Inspection of lower colon with a flexible scope. Patient may need to be sedated.
- **Small bowel follow-through (SBFT):** Used to detect abnormalities in the small intestine. Done in addition to a GI series.
- **Spinal tap:** See lumbar puncture.
- **Thallium:** Radionuclear dye used to assess heart functions.
- **Titer:** A blood test to determine the presence of antibodies.
- **Tuberculin skin test:** Test for tuberculosis using tuberculin purified protein derivative (PPD).
- **Ultrasonography:** Reflection of sound waves.
- **Venography:** Radiographic examination used to locate a thrombus in a vein.

For additional information on diagnostic testing and procedures, consult the following:

Pagana KD, Pagana TJ: *Mosby's manual of diagnostic and laboratory tests,* ed 6, St. Louis, 2018, Elsevier.

Pagana KD, Pagana TJ, Pagana TN: *Mosby's diagnostic and laboratory test reference,* ed 12, St. Louis, 2015, Mosby.

Perry AG, Potter PA, Ostendorf WR: *Clinical nursing skills and techniques,* ed 9, St. Louis, 2018, Elsevier.

Potter PA, Perry AG, Stockert PA, Hall AM: *Fundamentals of nursing*, ed 10, St. Louis, 2021, Elsevier..

Yoost BL, Crawford LR: *Fundamentals of nursing: active learning for collaborative practice*, ed 2, St. Louis, 2020, Elsevier.

CHAPTER 28

Preoperative and Postoperative Care

PREOPERATIVE TEACHING
Coughing and Deep Breathing

- Preoperative teaching allows the patient time to practice techniques that will be used in the postoperative period and give a return demonstration to show understanding of the techniques.
- Coughing and deep breathing can prevent postoperative lung complications, including atelectasis and pneumonia.
- Postoperative patients utilize coughing and deep breathing to expand the lungs and improve ventilation.
- The patient should be in an upright position if possible (Fowler or semi-Fowler).
- Techniques include:
  - Deep breaths are inhaled through the nose and exhaled through the mouth:
    - Rest the palms of the hands below the rib cage, with the middle fingers touching.
    - Take slow, deep breaths, inhaling through the nose.

- Feel the abdomen push against the hands. Keep the chest and shoulders still.
- Inhale as deeply as possible and hold that breath for 3 to 5 seconds.
- Exhale slowly through pursed lips, and stop exhaling when the middle fingers touch again.
- Perform each inhalation and exhalation three to five times before resting.
- Perform all of these steps 10 times every hour if possible.
- Pursed-lip exhalation:
  - Purse the lips as if to make a whistling sound (into an O shape) and then release the breath in a slow, controlled exhalation.
- Controlled cough:
  - If the patient has an abdominal or thoracic incision, provide a splint.
  - Take two deep breaths in and out.
  - Then inhale as deeply as possible and hold it for 3 to 5 seconds.
  - Release the breath as a full cough; cough two or three times, but do not inhale between coughs if possible.
  - Perform these steps two or three times every 2 hours if possible.

Incentive Spirometry
- Teaching a patient to use an incentive spirometer can prevent postoperative lung complications, including atelectasis and pneumonia, because it encourages deep inhalation.
- The patient attempts to reach a set inhalation volume, which may be set by the primary care provider or respiratory therapy specialist or calculated from standardized charts.

- The patient should be in an upright position (semi-Fowler or Fowler) if possible.
- The goal is to have a steady rise of a marker in the device to achieve a specific inhalation volume, which is marked on the device.
- Instruct the patient to:
  - Inhale slowly and as much as possible with the mouth on the mouthpiece.
  - Hold that breath for 3 to 5 seconds.
  - Remove mouthpiece and exhale slowly.
  - Repeat each inhalation and exhalation 5 to 12 times.
  - End with two controlled coughs.
  - Perform this exercise every 1 to 2 hours per orders.

Leg Exercises
- Postoperative leg exercises are performed to encourage venous return, prevent deep vein thrombosis, and maintain joint mobility.
- Passive range of motion should be completed for patients who cannot accomplish active range of motion.
- Teach leg exercises in the preoperative period.
- Have the patient lie supine in bed.
  - Foot circles:
    - Rotate each foot at the ankle making a circle, first clockwise, then counterclockwise.
    - Perform five circles in each direction.
  - Dorsiflexion and plantar flexion:
    - Point the toes toward the foot of the bed, then point the toes toward the head as far as possible.
    - Repeat 5 times.

- Quadriceps setting:
  - With legs extended, tighten the thigh muscle and push the knee downward toward the mattress.
  - Hold for a few seconds then relax the leg.
  - Complete five sets on each leg.
- Leg raises:
  - Lift one leg up from the bed with the knee slightly flexed.
  - Continue lifting the leg while bending at the knee and the hip.
  - Bring the leg up as far as possible without discomfort.
  - Alternate legs and repeat 5 times on each side.

Splinting

- Postoperative splinting is used to support an incision and to promote comfort by decreasing pressure and pain related to an incision.
- Used during coughing, deep breathing, or movement that may cause sutures to pull or tear.
- Postoperative splinting is used primarily for incision sites on the abdomen and the thorax.
- One of the patient's hands is placed on top of the incision; the other hand is placed on top of the first, applying slight pressure.
- For comfort, the patient may use a pillow, holding it under the hands and over the incision.
- After placement, the patient may continue with controlled coughing and deep-breathing procedures or with movement, such as repositioning in bed or transferring out of bed.

PREOPERATVE CHECKLIST

	Initials
Preoperative Data	
Height _____ Weight _____	
Isolation Y or N Type _____	
Allergies noted on chart Y or N	
Vital signs (baseline) T ____ P ____ R ____ BP ____ Pulse Ox ____	
Chart Review	
H&P on chart	
H&P within 30 days? Y or N	
Signed and witnessed informed consent form on chart Y or N	
Signed consent for blood administration Y or NA	
Blood type and crossmatch Y or NA	
Diagnostic Results	
Hgb/Hct ____ / ____ NA	
PT/INR/PTT ____ / ____ / ____ NA	

Continued

PREOPERATVE CHECKLIST—Cont'd

Preoperative Data	Initials
CXR _____ NA	
ECG _____ NA	
hCG _____ Negative _____ Positive _____ NA	
Other labs:	
Final Chart Review	
Additional forms attached:	
Day of Surgery	
Surgical site marked Y or NA	
ID band on patient Y or N	
Allergy band on patient Y or NA	
Vital signs Time _____	
T _____ P _____ R _____ BP _____ Pulse Ox _____	

PREOPERATVE CHECKLIST—Cont'd

Preoperative Data	Initials
Procedures	
NPO since _____	
Capillary blood glucose Time _____ Result: _____ NA	
Voided/catheter Time _____	
Preoperative drugs given	
Time _____ NA	
Preoperative antibiotics given	
Time _____ NA	
Preoperative skin prep Y or NA	
Shower_____ Scrub_____ Clip_____	
Makeup, nail polish, false fingernails, and false eyelashes removed Y or NA	
Hospital gown applied Y or NA	
Valuables	

Continued

PREOPERATVE CHECKLIST—Cont'd

Preoperative Data	Initials
Dentures Y or N	
Wig or hairpiece Y or N	
Eyeglasses Y or N	
Contact lenses Y or N	
Hearing aid Y or N	
Prosthesis Y or N	
Jewelry Y or N Piercings with jewelry Y or N	
Clothing Y or N	
Disposition of valuables: Hearing aid in place Y or NA	
Time to OR _____ Date _____	
Transported to OR by _____	
Final check by _____ RN _____	

From Lewis SL, Bucher L, Heitkemper MM, et al: *Medical-surgical nursing*, ed 10, St. Louis, 2017, Elsevier.

POSTOPERATIVE NURSING CARE
Postanesthesia Care Unit (PACU)

- Provides a safe environment for the patient to be monitored during the immediate postoperative period.
- The PACU nurse is trained to prevent potential complication and react quickly when complications arise.
- Handoff report from the surgical nurse to the PACU nurse should include:
  - Type of surgery and anesthetic
  - Findings and results of the surgery
  - Complications during the surgery
  - Transfusions given during surgery
  - Current respiratory status of the patient
  - Current cardiac and circulatory status of the patient
  - Types and number of incisions, drains, tubes, and IV lines
  - Current vital signs and when they need to be taken next
  - Current laboratory values and when specimens need to be drawn next
  - Dressing location, condition, and changes. Note that the first change is generally done by the surgeon.
  - Neurological status and need for future neurological checks
  - Time, frequency, and route of administration of pain medications
  - Additional postoperative orders
  - Whether family or significant others are waiting for the patient
- The PACU nurse assesses the patient immediately after transfer and at specified intervals during the time in the PACU.

- Care in the PACU includes:
  - Airway management
  - Monitoring vital signs
  - Monitoring neurological status
  - Pain management
  - Wound or dressing assessment
  - IV fluid management
- Certain criteria must be met before the patient is discharged from the PACU to a nursing unit. Standardized scores are used, such as the Aldrete score or the postanesthesia recovery score (PARS), which rate the patient's vital signs, level of consciousness, respiratory status, and activity.

Nursing Unit

- Patients who meet discharge criteria from the PACU may go to a surgical nursing unit.
- Unstable patients may be transferred to an intensive care unit.
- Handoff report from the PACU nurse to the unit nurse should include all of the information listed under PACU handoff.
- In addition, the PACU nurse updates the patient's current status.
- The unit nurse assesses the patient immediately after transfer and at frequent intervals depending on the surgery and the patient's status.
- Postoperative orders are intended to prevent complications, and nursing care may include:
  - Early ambulation
  - Fluids and hydration
  - Diet advancement with the return of peristalsis
  - Wound care
  - Leg exercises
  - Coughing and deep breathing
  - Incentive spirometer
  - Pain management

Postoperative Complications

- Postoperative nursing care is focused on prevention of complications, close monitoring of the patient, and immediate response to changes in the patient's condition.
- Airway obstruction
  - **Causes:** Tongue blocking the airway, laryngospasms, bronchospasms, aspiration.
  - **Signs and symptoms:** Difficulty breathing; decreased respiration or breath sounds; loud, crowing sound as the patient attempts to breathe.
  - **Nursing interventions:** Depending on the underlying cause, an anesthesia team member may need to be consulted immediately for reintubation. Other interventions include repositioning the patient, manual opening of the airway, removal of obstruction, manual resuscitation with an ambu bag.
- Hemorrhage
  - **Causes:** Weak sutures, stress on the surgical site, medications, a clot that has dislodged, internal bleeding.
  - **Signs and symptoms:** Obvious bright red blood from the incision; increased, weak, thready pulse; tachypnea; hypotension; pale, cold, clammy skin; anxiety; restlessness; thirst; decreased urine output.
  - **Nursing interventions:** Monitor blood pressure, heart rate, rhythm, quality; assess for bleeding; apply pressure to external bleeding sites; alert the surgical team and/or rapid response team depending on the patient's condition.
- Shock
  - **Causes:** Hemorrhage in the postoperative period, severe hypovolemia, sepsis.

- **Signs and symptoms:** Hypotension, rapid heart rate, decreased capillary refill, rapid, shallow breathing, nausea, vomiting, restlessness followed by lethargy, pale to mottled skin, cold and clammy, dry mucus membranes.
- **Nursing intervention:** Maintain patent patient airway; administer oxygen as ordered; assess vital signs, oxygen saturation, skin color, level of consciousness, and urine output; obtain or maintain IV access; elevate patient's feet while keeping head flat or minimally elevated; examine for obvious loss of blood; follow facility protocols for intravenous fluid and drug administration; remain with patient while activating rapid response team or facility protocol for shock.
- Thrombophlebitis
  - **Causes:** Immobility during or after surgery.
  - **Signs and symptoms:** Red, warm, edematous leg or calf; pain in the lower leg.
  - **Nursing intervention:** Check for leg tenderness and edema. Preventative measures include: leg exercises, early ambulation if appropriate, TED hose and sequential compression devices while in bed; administer anticoagulants as ordered.
- Pulmonary Embolism
  - **Causes:** Immobility, deep vein thrombosis, or venous thromboembolism.
  - **Signs and symptoms:** Sudden onset chest pain that increases with deep inspiration, shortness of breath, anxiety, restlessness, dry cough, hemoptysis, dyspnea, cyanosis, diaphoresis. Additional symptoms may include hypotension, hypoxemia, tachypnea, and loss of consciousness.

- **Nursing intervention:** Alert the rapid response team or equivalent in your facility; assist alert patients to sit up as high as possible to facilitate air exchange; administer oxygen per facility policy and follow prescribed facility treatment protocol.
- Pneumonia
  - **Causes:** Aspiration, excess pulmonary secretions, immobility, failure to cough deeply, depression of the cough reflex.
  - **Signs and symptoms:** Dyspnea, adventitious breath sounds, chest pain, chills, fever, productive cough.
  - **Nursing interventions:** Encourage use of incentive spirometer, nebulizer treatments, administer antibiotic therapy and other medications as ordered, sitting position if possible, hydration, oxygen administration.
- Atelectasis
  - **Causes:** Airways blocked with secretions.
  - **Signs and symptoms:** Cough, dyspnea, anxiety, chest pain, cyanosis, diminished breath sounds over the affected area, crackles.
  - **Nursing interventions:** Focused on prevention: assess vital signs and oxygen saturation; assess lungs; turn patient every 1 to 2 hours unless contraindicated or encourage ambulation if allowed; have patient cough and deep breathe using pillows to splint incisions every 1 to 2 hours; have patient use incentive spirometer as ordered every 1 to 2 hours; provide adequate hydration; administer pain medications; early ambulation. Focused on treatment: Use humidification to ease breathing; perform chest therapy, if ordered, to help thin secretions and postural drainage to drain

secretions; suction if necessary; oxygen administration if ordered.

- Wound complications
  - **Nursing interventions**: Focus on preventing wound complications following surgery. Wounds are kept clean with appropriate dressings. Stress on the wound is reduced by having the patient splint the wound when moving or coughing.
  - Infection
    - **Causes:** Bacteria entering the incision either in the operating room or during wound care.
    - **Signs and symptoms:** Red, warm-draining, foul-smelling wound.
    - **Nursing interventions:** Wound care as ordered; administer antibiotics as ordered.
- Dehiscence
  - **Causes:** Pressure on the incision from sneezing, coughing, vomiting, or movement; removal of the sutures before the incision is healed; obesity.
  - **Signs and symptoms:** Separation of the edges of the incision; large amount of serosanguinous fluid on the dressing.
  - **Nursing interventions:** Place the patient in Fowler or semi-Fowler position; cover the wound with a sterile saline dressing; notify the surgeon immediately.
- Evisceration
  - **Causes:** Pressure on the incision from sneezing, coughing, vomiting, or movement; removal of the sutures before the incision is healed; obesity.
  - **Signs and symptoms:** Separation of the edges of the incision with protrusion of organs through the incision; large amount of serosanguinous fluid on the dressing.
  - **Nursing interventions:** Place the patient in Fowler or semi-Fowler position; cover the

wound with a sterile saline dressing; notify the surgeon immediately.

- Genitourinary: loss of voluntary control over the bladder
  - **Causes:** Anesthesia.
  - **Signs and symptoms:** Difficulty voiding after surgery or after catheter is removed.
  - **Nursing interventions:** Encourage adequate fluid intake; assess I & O; monitor for bladder distention; assess the need for and care of Foley catheter or need for straight catheterization.
- Gastrointestinal: impaired or absent peristalsis
  - **Causes:** Anesthesia; manipulation of the bowels during abdominal surgery.
  - **Signs and symptoms:** Nausea; faint or absent bowel sounds.
  - **Nursing interventions:** Assess bowel sounds for possible ileus, indicated by absent bowel sounds. Assess for nausea, vomiting, distended abdomen, and gas pains. Advance diet only after the return of peristalsis.

For additional information on preoperative and postoperative care, consult the following:

Ignatavicius DD, Workman ML, Rebar CR: *Medical-surgical nursing: patient-centered collaborative care,* ed 9, St. Louis, 2018, Elsevier.

Lewis SL, Bucher L, Heitkemper MM, et al: *Medical-surgical nursing,* ed 10, St. Louis, 2017, Elsevier.

Perry AG, Potter PA, Ostendorf WR: *Clinical nursing skills and techniques,* ed 9, St. Louis, 2018, Elsevier.

Phillips N: *Berry and Kohn's operating room technique,* ed 13, St. Louis, 2017, Elsevier.

Potter PA, Perry AG, Stockert PA, Hall AM: *Fundamentals of nursing,* ed 10, St. Louis, 2021, Elsevier.

Rothrock JC, McEwen DR: *Alexander's care of the patient in surgery,* ed 16, St. Louis, 2019, Elsevier.

Yoost BL, Crawford LR: *Fundamentals of nursing: active learning for collaborative practice,* ed 2, St. Louis, 2020, Elsevier.

CHAPTER 29

Emergent Clinical Situations

MYOCARDIAL INFARCTION (MI)

- **Signs and symptoms**
  - Chest pain or a squeezing, crushing, or heavy feeling in the chest, shortness of breath, dyspnea, lightheadedness, stomach pain or pressure, pain in left arm, back, or in the neck or jaw, diaphoresis, nausea, fatigue
- **Causes**
  - Blockage of one or more coronary arteries secondary to plaque buildup
- **Nursing Intervention**
  - Alert the Rapid Response Team or equivalent in your facility.
  - Follow facility protocol to ensure patient safety and initiate required care.

CARDIAC ARREST
- **Signs and symptoms**
  - Loss of cardiac function, loss of consciousness
- **Causes**
  - Electrical disruption leading to lack of blood flow to vital organs
- **Nursing interventions**
  - Call a code consistent with facility policy.
  - Position patient in flat supine position.
  - Initiate CPR and continue until code team arrives.
  - Ask visitors to wait in the reception area (if consistent with facility protocol).

PULMONARY EMBOLISM
- **Signs and symptoms**
  - Sudden onset chest pain that increases with deep inspiration, shortness of breath, dry cough, hemoptysis, dyspnea, cyanosis, diaphoresis. Additional symptoms may include hypotension, hypoxemia, and loss of consciousness.
- **Causes**
  - Immobility, deep vein thrombosis, or venous thromboembolism.
- **Nursing intervention.**
  - Alert rapid response team or equivalent in your facility.
  - Assist alert patients to sit up as high as possible to facilitate air exchange.
  - Administer oxygen per facility policy and follow prescribed facility treatment protocol.

STROKE
- **Signs and symptoms**
  - Difficulty speaking, paralysis or loss of feeling in the extremities or face, sudden onset of severe headache, blurred vision, unsteady gait.

- **Causes**
  - Ischemia secondary to thrombus, or plaque blocking a brain artery, or embolus moving from its origin to an artery supplying blood to the brain.
  - Hemorrhage secondary to a blood vessel leakage or rupture.
- **Nursing interventions**
  - Alert the rapid response team or equivalent in your facility.
  - Be prepared for patient transfer to intensive care unit for immediate CAT scan and intervention based on cause of the stroke.
- Helpful Acronym for Patient Teaching: **FAST**
  - **F**ace—Is there a facial droop?
  - **A**rms—Does one arm drift downward when both are raised?
  - **S**peech—Is speech slurred or incoherent?
  - **T**ime—Call 9-1-1 immediately to initiate care as quickly as possible.

HYPERGLYCEMIA

- **Signs and symptoms**
  - "Warm and dry, sugar's high," increased thirst, headache, fatigue, impaired vision.
  - Blood sugar level ≥200mg/dL.
- **Causes**
  - Impaired production of insulin by the pancreas or diminished effectiveness of insulin to maintain blood glucose levels within normal range.
  - Increased levels of circulating blood glucose.
- **Nursing interventions**
  - Monitor vital signs, intake and output, and blood glucose levels.
  - Administer insulin as prescribed.
  - Document hyperglycemic episode and notify primary care provider (PCP).

HYPOGLYCEMIA
- **Signs and symptoms**
  - "Cold and clammy, eat some candy," jittery, diaphoretic, hungry, tired, dizzy, pale, confused.
  - Blood sugar level <70 mg/dL.
- **Causes**
  - Increased physical exercise, illness, skipping meals, inadequate carbohydrate intake.
  - Too much insulin or oral antihyperglycemic medication.
- **Nursing interventions**
  - Supply patient, who is not NPO, with 15 to 20 grams of glucose or simple carbohydrates, which may include:
    - Orange or apple juice, 4-6 ounces
    - Glucose tablets
    - Sugar packet
    - Hard candy or the equivalent
  - Check blood glucose level in 15 minutes following carbohydrate ingestion.
  - Administer glucagon per facility policy if blood glucose levels do not return to normal range after two ingestions of simple carbohydrate followed by blood glucose testing.
  - Document hypoglycemic episode and notify PCP.

SEIZURES
- **Signs and symptoms**
  - Staring, involuntary jerking of extremities, decreased or complete loss of consciousness, repetitive movements with lack of awareness.
- **Causes**
  - Elevated body temperature, increased intracranial pressure, hyponatremia, brain tumors, use of recreational drugs, alcohol abuse,

medication reactions, head trauma, epilepsy, genetic predisposition.
- **Nursing interventions**
  - Place patients with a history of seizures on seizure precautions upon admission:
    - Pad bed siderails; keep an oral airway and suctioning equipment at the bedside.
    - Do not place anything in the patient's mouth during seizure activity.
  - Protect patient from harm throughout a seizure.
  - Follow facility protocol regarding specific treatment.
  - Document seizure activity and notify PCP.

See Chapter 18 for additional information on seizure precautions.

SHOCK
- **Signs and symptoms**
  - Hypotension, rapid heart rate, decreased capillary refill, rapid and shallow breathing, nausea, vomiting, restlessness followed by lethargy, pale to mottled skin, cold and clammy, dry mucus membranes.
- **Causes**
  - Hemorrhage, severe hypovolemia, anaphylaxis, sepsis, neural or chemical dysfunction, severe emotional trauma.
- **Nursing interventions**
  - Maintain patent patient airway.
  - Administer oxygen as ordered.
  - Assess vital signs, oxygen saturation, skin color, level of consciousness, and urine output.
  - Obtain or maintain IV access.
  - Elevate patient's feet while keeping head flat or minimally elevated.
  - Examine for obvious loss of blood.

- Follow facility protocols for intravenous fluid and drug administration.
- Remain with patient while activating rapid response team or facility protocol for shock.

SUICIDE POTENTIAL
- **Signs and symptoms**
  - Verbalizes or demonstrates cues of interest and potential for committing suicide, giving possessions away, withdrawing from friends or family.
- **Risk Factors**
  - Depression, isolation, suicidal ideation with a plan, history of child abuse, family history of suicide, hopelessness, psychiatric or medical illness, unemployment, aggressiveness, alcohol or drug abuse, imminent incarceration, sexual orientation concerns, impulsivity, high-stress profession.
- **Nursing interventions**
  - Assess for risk factors.
  - Observe if the patient has recently become happy after having been depressed.
  - Provide environmental protection, as needed,
  - Ask patients if they have a plan; if so, initiate suicide precautions.
  - Refer for professional counseling.

For additional information on emergent clinical situations, consult the following:

Ignatavicius D, Workman M, Blair M, et al: *Medical-surgical nursing: patient-centered collaborative care,* ed 9, St. Louis, 2018, Elsevier.
Lewis S, Bucher L, Heitkemper M, et al: *Medical-surgical nursing,* ed 10, St. Louis, 2017, Elsevier.
Potter PA, Perry AG, Stockert PA, Hall AM: *Fundamentals of nursing,* ed 10, St. Louis, 2021, Elsevier.

Halter M: *Varcarolis' foundations of psychiatric mental health nursing: a clinical approach,* ed 8, St. Louis, 2018, Elsevier.

Yoost BL, Crawford LR: *Fundamentals of nursing: active learning for collaborative practice,* ed 2, St. Louis, 2020, Elsevier.

CHAPTER 30

Death and Dying

LEGAL TERMINOLOGY RELATED TO DEATH

Advance Directives

- Living will
  - A document specifying the treatment a person wants to receive when he or she is unconscious or no longer capable of making decisions independently.
  - May address end-of-life care and the circumstances under which treatment should be withheld or stopped.
  - May also address when a person wants to have extraordinary measures, such as ventilator assistance for breathing, terminated.
- Durable power of attorney
  - Legal document that designates a person to make legal decisions on behalf of another person who is unable to make independent decisions.

- Limits are set on the power that the designated person has.
- Decisions are not limited to medical care.
- Most commonly a spouse, parent, child, or other close relative is the designated power of attorney.
- Healthcare proxy
  - Specific durable power of attorney for health care.
  - A legal document that specifies the person who can make medical decisions for an individual who is unable to comprehend information or communicate.
  - Limited power of attorney that covers health care and treatment decisions.
  - Alternate proxies may be named in the event that the primary proxy is unavailable.

Coroner's Case
- The coroner is notified of any death that is a homicide; suicide; accidental, sudden, or suspicious death.
- The coroner makes the decision, based on information reported, whether a death warrants a postmortem medical examination.
- Each state has different laws regarding what type of death qualifies as a coroner's case.

Death Certificate
- The legal document that identifies the date, location, time, and cause(s) of death.

Do-Not-Resuscitate (DNR) Orders
- Orders that outline the patient's desire to refuse or limit treatment.
- DNR terminology may vary by state. Be familiar with the terms used in your state.

- Examples of different DNR orders:
  - Do-not-resuscitate (DNR): a person will not receive CPR if cardiac or respiratory arrest occurs.
  - Do-not-resuscitate-comfort care only (DNR-CCO): a person will not receive CPR but will receive interventions that make the patient more comfortable, such as pain medication, complimentary therapy to relieve pain, emotional support, and hygienic care, whether or not cardiac or respiratory arrest occurs.
  - Do-not-resuscitate-comfort care arrest (DNR-CCA): the person can receive lifesaving medications and treatments if cardiac or respiratory arrest has not occurred. If the person arrests, only comfort care will be provided.
- Health care facilities should make sure that the wishes of the person and family are being carried out completely and correctly.

Establishing the Time of Death
- Time of death occurs and is documented when there is absence of heart rate, blood pressure, respiration, pupillary reflexes, and response to external stimuli.

Final Disposition
- Final destination for the body.
- The hospital morgue, county morgue, or funeral home is generally the final disposition of the body.

Hospice
- The hospice interdisciplinary health care team provides comfort and supportive care for terminally ill patients and their families.
- Care can be in the patient's home, in the hospital, in another health care facility, or in a specialized hospice facility.

- Curative care is no longer offered.
- Goal of care is symptom control and comfort measures.

Palliative Care
- Patients are not terminally ill but need high-quality symptom control for a serious or life-threatening illness.
- Appropriate for anyone who has a chronic, debilitating condition.
- Improves the patient's quality of life.
- Provides relief from pain and other distressing symptoms.
- Palliative care may include curative care.
- It is used in conjunction with other therapies that are intended to prolong life, such as chemotherapy or radiation therapy, and includes those interventions needed to manage distressing clinical complications.

Persistent Vegetative State
- A condition when a patient is unresponsive to verbal, physical, or psychological stimuli and shows no signs of cognitive function.
- Usually the patient is being kept alive through medical interventions such as Intravenous therapy, tube feedings, ventilator assistance, etc.

Postmortem or Autopsy
- A medical examination conducted after death by a pathologist, forensic pathologist, or county coroner to determine the exact cause of death.

Pronouncement
- The nurse identifies the patient; documents the absence of heart rate, blood pressure, respirations, reflexes, and response to external stimuli; notes the

time of death; and calls the appropriate medical professional, depending on the facility, to pronounce death.

- The nurse documents all of the above in the patient's electronic health record (EHR).
- Each state has practice guidelines that determine who can pronounce death.

STAGES OF DYING AND GRIEF*
Denial
- Patient or family may refuse to accept the situation.
- Patient or family may not believe the diagnosis.
- Patient or family may seek second and third opinions.
- Patient or family may claim that the test results were wrong.
- Patient or family may claim that the tests were mixed up with those of someone else.
- Patient may sleep more or be overly talkative or cheerful.

Anger
- Patient or family may be hostile.
- Patient or family may have excessive demands.
- Patient may be withdrawn, cold, or unemotional.
- Feelings may include envy, resentment, or rage.
- Patient may be angry at family for being well.
- Patient may be uncooperative or manipulative.
- This may be the time that patients are the hardest to care for but the time when they need us the most!

---

*From Kübler-Ross E: *On death and dying,* New York, 1969, Collier Books; and Kübler-Ross E: *Questions and answers on death and dying,* New York, 1974, Collier Books.

Bargaining
- Patient or family may promise to improve or change habits such as quit smoking, eat less, or exercise more.
- Bargaining may be intertwined with feelings of guilt.
- Bargains are often with the physicians or with God.

Depression
- Patient or family may speak of the upcoming loss.
- Patient or family may cry or weep often.
- Patient or family may want to be alone.

Acceptance
- Patient may exhibit a decreased interest in the surroundings.
- Patient may not want visitors during this time.
- Do not confuse acceptance with depression.
- There seems to be a calmness or peace about the patient.

NURSING INTERVENTIONS RELATED TO THE STAGES OF GRIEF
Denial
- Denial is used as a coping or protective function and should not be viewed as a bad quality. It can be a time when a patient or family can gather their thoughts, feelings, and strengths.
- Nursing interventions:
  - Educate the patient and family about the stages of grief.
  - Encourage exercise, rest, sleep, journaling, stress-relieving techniques, and other healthy coping mechanisms.
  - Listen to the patient and family; they may need an outlet to express their feelings.

- Refer the patient and family to community resources.
- Be open and honest with communications.
- Avoid giving false hope.
- Do not argue with the patient or family.

Anger
- Anger is often directed at caregivers.
- Nursing interventions:
  - Do not take anger personally.
  - Help the family realize they should not take anger personally.
  - Check on the patient often and answer call lights promptly.
  - Assist the family with much-needed breaks.

Bargaining
- Many people bargain with a higher power, therefore this may be a private phase.
- Nursing interventions:
  - Provide frequent chances for the patient or family to talk.
  - Offer to contact clergy, chaplain, or other support persons.

Depression
- Some patients or families may not have a good outlet for their depression.
- Nursing interventions:
  - Do not force cheerful or important conversation.
  - Allow the patient or family time to talk and voice concerns.
  - Offer to contact clergy or chaplain of the patient's choice.
  - Offer other cultural or religious support, as desired by the patient.

Acceptance
- Patient may want to be alone and families may feel rejected.
- Nursing interventions:
  - Encourage family to come often but for brief visits.
  - Offer to contact clergy or chaplain of the patient's choice.
  - Offer other cultural or religious support as desired or requested by the patient.

NURSING CARE FOR THE PATIENT WHO IS DYING
Assessment of the Dying Patient
- Signs and symptoms of impending death:
  - Decrease in urine output.
  - Cold, mottled extremities.
  - Decrease in blood pressure.
  - Decrease in heart rate.
  - Changes in breathing patterns with periods of apnea.
  - Respiratory congestion due to inability to handle secretions, "death rattle."

Personal Care
- Provide thorough, frequent mouth care; keep mouth moist using dampened toothettes.
- Bathe the patient and provide perineal care as needed.
- Use gentle massage if desired by the patient or family.
- Apply lip balm.
- Instill artificial tears if eyes are open and dry.
- Offer adequate pain control with medications, massage, and positioning.
- Suction, if there are increased secretions, to ease breathing.

- Clean and straighten linens often.
- Change the position of patient as needed to promote comfort and prevent pressure injuries.
- Provide adequate hydration.

Special Needs
- Encourage visits by clergy or chaplain of the patient's choice.
- Honor requests for Last Rites, Holy Communion, or other religious or cultural ceremonies.
- Allow for religious music, holy books, and other supports.
- Allow time for the family or friends to pray.
- Encourage cultural or religious rituals or practices.
- Urge families to bring comfort items such as photos, pillows, or other treasured momentos.
- Control symptoms to promote comfort and prevent undue suffering.

Caring for the Family
- Describe the physical changes that may be taking place as death approaches.
- Allow the family as much time as possible with the dying patient.
- Provide open and honest updates to the family about the signs of approaching death.
- Educate the family about care measures that are controlling symptoms or providing comfort for their loved one.
- Allow for sleep and hygiene needs of the family or friends.
- Let the family or friends voice fears or concerns.
- Allow the family time for questions.
- Encourage the family to express their emotions.

NURSING INTERVENTIONS AFTER DEATH

If the family is *not* present at the time of death:

- Assess for any special religious, cultural, or family instructions.
- Review the facility's policies and procedure for preparation.
- Assess for any legal limitations in preparing the body.
- Wear gloves when preparing the body.
- The body should be placed flat with the arms and legs straight.
- The eyes and mouth should be closed. Insert dentures if possible.
- Remove all intravenous lines, nasogastric tubes, Foley catheters, etc., unless the patient is going to have an autopsy. In cases where an autopsy is necessary as required by law or requested by family, all lines and tubes must remain in the body.
- Clean away any excretions and secretions.
- Dress the body in a clean gown, if possible.
- Brush the hair.
- Cover the body up to the chest with a clean sheet.
- Remove all soiled linens from the room.
- Position the body supine with the head elevated on a pillow, hand on top of the sheet.
- Remove all excess equipment and trash from room.
- Pack up all other personal items and label with the patient's name.
- Document nursing care and interventions in the patient's EHR and wait for the family.

If the family is present at the time of death:

- Allow the family time to be with their loved one.
- Ask the family if there are any religious or cultural rituals that need to be honored.
- Allow the family to assist with preparation of the body if they wish.

- Assist the family in packing up the belongings.
- Help the family with any paperwork.
- Allow the family to call other family members, if needed.
- Support the family in contacting a funeral home or making other arrangements.
- After the family has gone, prepare the body for removal per the facility's protocol. Usually this involves wrapping the body in a shroud, cloth, sheet, or bag for transportation to the morgue or funeral home. The body is identified by tags according to facility policy.
- Document nursing care and interventions in the patient's medical record.

HOSPICE CARE IN THE HOME*

- Patients receiving hospice in the home require skilled, knowledgeable nurses to provide a high level of care, because many needs are specific for the dying patient and the family of that patient. Care includes:
  - Assessment of safety in the home related to the physical as well as social environment.
  - Physical as well as psychosocial assessment conducted in an independent and thorough manner.
  - Coordination with all members of the health care team.
  - Assure that family members providing care are knowledgeable and able to provide the necessary physical care.
  - Safe use of equipment that is being used in the home and provision of necessary services.

---

*From Yoost BL, Crawford LR: Fundamentals of nursing: active learning for collaborative practice, ed 2, St. Louis, 2020, Elsevier.

ORGAN DONATION

- Consent for organ donation must be in writing with the individual's signature.
- In many states, even if there is signed consent, the family still has to give consent after death.
- The United Network for Organ Sharing (UNOS) establishes policies and procedures for obtaining and allocating donated organs to waiting recipients.
- Nurses need to be aware of facility policies and procedures for organ and tissue donation.
- Most facilities have special teams of professionals who are knowledgeable about organ donation and procurement. They should be contacted to talk with family members and to arrange for retrieval of organs and tissues.

For additional information on death and dying, consult the following:

Kuebler KK, Heidrich DE, Esper P: *Palliative and end-of-life care,* ed 2, St. Louis, 2007, Elsevier.

Perry AG, Potter PA, Ostendorf WR: *Clinical nursing skills and techniques,* ed 9, St. Louis, 2018, Elsevier.

Potter PA, Perry AG, Stockert PA, Hall AM: *Fundamentals of nursing,* ed 10, St. Louis, 2021, Elsevier.

Yoost BL, Crawford LR: *Fundamentals of nursing: active learning for collaborative practice,* ed 2, St. Louis, 2021, Elsevier.

Index

Note: Page numbers followed by *f* indicate figures and *t* indicate tables.